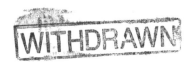

Springer Series on the Teaching of Nursing

Diane O. McGivern, RN, PhD, FAAN, Series Editor

2004   Developing An Online Course: Best Practices for Nurse Educators, *Carol A. O'Neil, PhD, RN, Cheryl A. Fisher, MSN, RN, Susan K. Newbold, RNBC, FAAN*

2004   Academic Nursing Practice: Helping to Shape the Future of Healthcare, *L. Evans, DNSc, FAAN, RN, Norma M. Lang, PhD, FAAN, FRCN, RN*

2003   Teaching Nursing in an Associate Degree Program, *Rita G. Mertig, MS, RNC, CNS*

2000   Nursing Informatics: Education for Practice, *B. Carty, RN, EdD*

2000   Distance Education in Nursing, *J. M. Novotny, PhD, RN*

2000   Community-Based Nursing Education: The Experiences of Eight Schools of Nursing, *P. S. Matteson, PhD, RNC*

2000   A Nuts-and-Bolts Approach to Teaching Nursing, 2nd ed., *V. Schoolcraft, RN, MS, PhD, and J. M. Novotny, PhD, RN*

1999   Clinical Teaching Strategies in Nursing, *K. B. Gaberson, PhD, RN, and M. H. Oermann, PhD, RN, FAAN*

1999   Integrating Community Service into Nursing Education: A Guide to Service-Learning, *P. A. Bailey, EdD, RN, CS, D. R. Carpenter, EdD, RN, CS, and P. Harrington, EdD, RN, CS*

1999   Teaching Nursing in the Era of Managed Care, *B. S. Barnum, RN, PhD, FAAN*

1998   Developing Research in Nursing and Health: Quantitative and Qualitative Methods, *C N. Hoskins, PhD, RN, FAAN*

1998   Evaluation and Testing in Nursing Education, *M. H. Oermann, PhD, RN, FAAN, and K. B. Gaberson, PhD, RN*

1996   Using the Arts and Humanities to Teach Nursing, *T. M. Valiga, RN, EdD, and E. R. Bruderle, MSN, RN*

1995   Teaching Nursing in the Neighborhoods: The Northeastern University Model, *P. S. Matteson, PhD, RNC*

1994   The Nurse As Group Leader: Third Edition, *C. C. Clark, EdD, RN, ARNP, FAAN*

1993   A Down-to-Earth Approach to Being a Nurse Educator, *V. Schoolcraft, RN, MS, PhD*

1993   An Addictions Curriculum for Nurses and Other Helping Professionals: Vols. I and II, *E. M. Burns, RN, PhD, FAAN, A. Thompson, RN, PhD, and J. K. Ciccone, MA, APR, Editors*

1991   The Nurse Educator in Academia: Strategies for Success, *T. M. Valiga, RN, EdD, and H. J. Streubert, RN, EdD*

1990   Educating RNs for the Baccalaureates: Programs and Issues, *B. K. Redman, RN, PhD, and J. M. Cassells, MSN, DNSc*

1989   A Nuts-and-Bolts Approach to Teaching Nursing, *V. Schoolcraft, RN, MS, PhD*

Carol O'Neil, PhD, RN, is an Assistant Professor at the University of Maryland School of Nursing. Dr. O'Neil is a Web Initiative in Teaching (WIT) Fellow. Dr. O'Neil teaches online and has presented her research and experiences in teaching and learning online at both international and national conferences.

Cheryl Fisher, MSN, RN, is the Informatics/E-learning Manager for the Nursing Department at the National Institutes of Health (NIH). She has over 20 years experience at NIH, including positions with the National Heart Lung and Blood Institute. She works closely with nurse educators developing and delivering online educational offerings and managing the NIH Nursing Internet and Intranet Web sites. She also teaches Informatics for the University of Maryland and Nursing Theory and Nursing Research for the University of Phoenix Online. Currently she is enrolled at Towson University in Towson, Maryland as a doctoral student in instructional technology.

Susan K. Newbold, MS, RNBC, FAAN, is a healthcare informatics consultant and an online instructor for the graduate nursing program at Excelsior College in Albany, New York. She is certified in Nursing Informatics by the American Nurses Credentialing Center. Ms. Newbold has made over 165 presentations on healthcare informatics in the United States, Singapore, New Zealand, Australia, Canada, Brazil, Japan, and Sweden. She is the co-founder of CARING, an international nursing informatics special interest group. Ms. Newbold has numerous publications to her credit including coediting two editions of *Nursing Informatics: Where Caring and Technology Meet.*

DEVELOPING AN ONLINE COURSE
BEST PRACTICES FOR NURSE EDUCATORS

Carol A. O'Neil, PhD, RN
Cheryl A. Fisher, MSN, RN
Susan K. Newbold, MSN, RNBC, FAAN

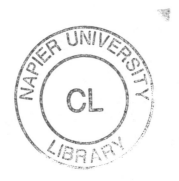

 ***Springer Series on the
Teaching of Nursing***

Springer Publishing Company, Inc.
536 Broadway
New York, NY 10012-3955

Acquisitions Editor: Ruth Chasek
Production Editor: Sally Ahearn
Cover design by Joanne Honigman

01 02 03 04 05 / 5 4 3 2 1

Library of Congress Cataloging-in-Publication-Data

O'Neil, Carol A.
    Developing an online course : best practices for nurse educators / Carol
A. O'Neil, Cheryl A. Fisher, Susan K. Newbold.
        p. ; cm. — (Teaching of nursing)
    Includes bibliographical references and index.
    ISBN 0-8261-2546-8
    1. Nursing—Study and teaching. 2. Internet in education.
[DNLM: 1. Education, Nursing—methods. 2. Internet. 3. Curriculum. 4.
Education, Distance. WY 18 O58d 2004] I. Fisher, Cheryl A. II. Newbold,
Susan K. III. Title. IV. Springer series on the teaching of nursing
(Unnumbered)
RT73.O59 2004
610.73'071'1—dc22   2004002041

Printed in the United States of America by Integrated Book Technology.

Contents

Acknowledgments	*vii*
Preface	*ix*
1 Introduction to Web-Based Teaching and Learning	1
2 Theories of Learning and the Online Environment	13
3 Developing the Infrastructure for Online Learning: Student, Faculty, and Technical Support	27
4 Technologies and Competencies Needed for Online Learning	47
5 Reconceptualizing the Online Course	59
6 Designing the Online Learning Environment	79
7 Course Management Methods	97
8 Interacting and Communicating Online	125
9 Assessment and Evaluation of Online Learning	137
Index	*165*

Acknowledgments

The authors acknowledge their colleagues at the University of Maryland School of Nursing for their inspiration, forward thinking, and support.

Preface

CAROL A. O'NEIL

The original purpose of the Web was to communicate and share information, and its development has dramatically changed our methods of communication and sharing information. Ultimately, it has changed the practice of nursing.

For one, it has spurred the growth of Nursing Informatics, which is defined by the American Nurses Association (ANA) as a specialty that integrates nursing science, computer science, and information science to manage and communicate data, information, and knowledge in nursing practice. Further, Nursing Informatics facilitates this integration to support patients, nurses, and other providers in their decision-making in all roles and settings. This support is accomplished through the use of information technology and information structures, which organize data, information, and knowledge for processing by computers. An international definition was adopted at the 1998 meeting of the International Medical Informatics Association Workgroup on Nursing Informatics in Seoul, Korea: Nursing Informatics is the integration of nursing, its information, and information management with information processing and communication technology, to support the health of people worldwide (Newbold, 2001).

While informatics focuses on interpreting databases, computers and the Web are used for additional purposes. As Internet Service Providers (ISP) such as America Online developed and refined their services, resources allowed for disseminating information and enhancing communication. Web sites such as Web-MD (Webmd.com), which advertises that it has 16 million users every month, were developed to provide information about health to the public. On-line "Ask-a-Nurse" sites are available for the public to get answers to specific questions about health. This method of imparting health information is called "Tele-Medicine" and is a growing area for nurses to practice.

Hospitals are developing in-house Websites (intranets). Information is disseminated by departments and nurse administrators who know how to develop and maintain intranet sites and who have a presence on the Web site. Training and certification is becoming fully or partially provided on the Web by continuing education departments, private continuing education companies, and other vendors. Meeting agendas may be developed through e-mail and meeting minutes can be distributed online. Meetings can be held online in virtual chat rooms, or live through cameras and voice streaming. The traditional 'go-somewhere-where-the-weather-is-beau-tiful-and-the-sun-is-shining' three-day conference is moving online. Conference presentations can be live or can be recorded before the conference. Keeping abreast of current trends in nursing and keep-ing connected to peers is facilitated through electronic mailing lists. For example, the Nursing Informatics CARING electronic mailing list under the management of Susan K. Newbold, MS, RN, FAAN includes over 840 subscribers.

The biggest area affected by the Web is in formal teaching environments as a result of online, Web-based classes in institu-tions of higher learning. The focus of this book is for nurses who are developing online health education and information for health consumers and professional peers and students. This may include:

- developing online courses in nursing education
- developing health education information Websites
- developing training or certification programs to enhance knowledge or skills

This book is about using computers in ways that expand the field of Nursing Informatics. It is about using the Web to teach student nurses, to train or retrain nurses, to certify competencies and skills, and to communicate. The nurse performing these activ-ities needs a set of knowledge and skills such as: pedagogy, the study of learning and specifically learning through a guided constructivist model (Chapter 2); the infrastructure needed to facilitate online strategies (Chapter 3); the technology hardware, software and courseware needed to teach and communicate in online environments (Chapter 4); reconceptualizing learning material from face-to-face to online environments (Chapter 5) and designing online learning environments (Chapter 6); managing online learning (Chapter 7); communicating and interacting (synchronous and asynchronous) (Chapter 8); and assessing and evaluating the impact of designs on learning and communicating (Chapter 9).

This book is about using the Web to impart information and to communicate. Therefore, teaching and learning in online environments is the focus of much of the discussion. However, keep in mind that many of the skills needed to teach nursing students are the same skills needed to develop a hospital intranet or an online conference.

REFERENCES

Newbold, S.K. (2001). A New Definition for Nursing Informatics. Underlying Nursing Practice, Administration, Education, and Research. *Advance for Nurses Online Edition.* Retrieved January 1, 2003, from *http://www.advancefornurses.com/CE_Tests/Informatics.html*

1

Introduction to Web-Based Teaching and Learning

Web-based instruction is an innovative approach for delivering information to a remote audience using the World Wide Web as the medium of delivery (Khan, 1997). Web-based learning reduces time and space barriers to learning and thus is called "anytime, anywhere learning". Instruction via the Web can be "technology enhanced" whereby technology enhances the learning process, or "technology delivered" whereby learning experiences are Web-based. Technology enhanced instruction may include traditional classroom experiences whereas, technology delivered instruction has no face-to-face meetings with the instructor/moderator and the learning experience is online. Instruction via the Web also includes "hybrid" or blended models of teaching (Young, 2002). A hybrid course is one in which some face-to-face learning experiences are replaced by virtual learning experiences or technology enhanced strategies.

Online instruction is instructor moderated, instructor taught, instructor mentored, yet student self-directed. There can be large discussion groups, small group discussions, individual activities, group activities, student-faculty/mentor interaction and student-student interaction. Material can be presented in a variety of ways including videotaping, audio taping, films, links to outside learning environment Web sites, charts, graphs, statistical data, formulas, and case studies. Interaction can be synchronous (real time) or asynchronous (delayed). Synchronous interaction means having a discussion by typing instead of talking. Asynchronous communication entails leaving messages at a specific posting site that others in the learning environment can read at their convenience. Individual courses, groups of courses, and entire programs are offered online. The degree of use of the Web in a course can range from the Web supplementing classroom learning, a mix of traditional classroom activities and online activities, to courses and programs that are offered completely online.

Online learners can be from traditional universities, such as Pennsylvania State University (*www.worldcampus.psu.edu*), or from virtual universities, such as California Virtual University (*www.california.edu* or *www.cvc.edu*). In addition to online courses and programs, there are online journals that focus on teaching and learning in online environments such as Journal of Asynchronous Learning Networks (*www.aln.org/alnweb/journal/jaln.htm*) or Education Review Technology Source at the University of North Carolina (*www.horizon.unc.edu/ts*). There are also professional groups for online teaching and learning such as Educause (*www.educause.edu*). The Center for Adult Learning purports that:

> Developments in technology and communications have brought about dramatic changes in both the learning needs and the way learning opportunities are delivered in business, labor, government, and academia. We are becoming a society in which continuous learning is central to effective participation as citizens and wage earners. Telecommunications technologies are not only transforming our needs for education and training, but they are expanding our capacity to respond to these needs. Distance learning, with a long history of serving isolated and remote learners, has now emerged as an effective, mainstream method of education and training that provides learning opportunities that are flexible and responsive to learners' needs. Distance learning is now a key component of our new learning society, in which learners must take increased responsibility for control and direction of the learning process (American Council on Education, n.d.).

There is no dispute that offering courses online is timely. But the question to be answered is how effective is it in student learning.

Thomas Russell at North Carolina State University studied hundreds of sources of written material about distance education (Russell, 1998) and concluded that the learning outcomes of students in the traditional classroom are similar to the learning outcomes of students in distance technology classes. Thus, the no significant differences phenomenon. The American Federation of Teachers and the National Education Association commissioned The Institute of Higher Education Policy "to conduct a review of the current research on the effectiveness of distance education, to analyze what the research tells us and does not tell us" (Merisotis & Phipps, 1999). Merisotis and Phipps (1999) conducted the review of the studies published from 1990 to present and the resultant document is called "What's the Difference: A Review of Contemporary Research on the Effectiveness of Distance Learning in Education." Overall, students online tended to perform as effectively as traditional students. Online students had similar learning experiences and were as satisfied with their learning experience as traditional students. But the authors noted several shortcomings in the original research: lack of control for extraneous variables; lack of randomization of subjects; questionable validity and reliability of instruments used to measure student outcome and attitude; no control for reactive effects such as the impact of motivation and interest because taking a course online is a novelty. The authors suggest that because of these shortcomings, the conclusions are inconclusive. The question that prevails is "What is the best way to teach students?" (Merisotis & Phipps, 1999, p. 17).

Chickering and Ehrman (1996) used the American Association for Higher Educations' (AAHE) Principles for Good Practice to develop best practices to teach students in online environments in a paper called "Implementing the Seven Principles: Technology as Lever". They suggest the following:

1. Good practice encourages contact between students and faculty: asynchronous communication (time delayed) is enhanced by using online environments. Students and faculty exchange work more effectively and safely in online environments than in the traditional classroom. Communication becomes more intimate, protected and connected online than in face-to-face interaction.

2. Good practice develops reciprocity and cooperation among students: technology provides opportunities for interaction in online learning environments. Students can share their knowledge and experience in small groups, study groups, during group problem solving and in activities related to learning content. For example, the learning content may be epidemiology and the epidemiologic triangle: the agent, the host, and the environment. Online students can be assigned to small learning groups and given the assignment, "Explain how West Nile virus occurs and develop strategies to prevent it from occurring."

3. Good practice uses active learning techniques: the technology included in online learning systems provides opportunity for active learning. For example, students in an online community health nursing course are given an exercise to assess a community. Students are directed to obtain census and vital statistics data. Students then view a windshield survey (made by faculty). The exercise is to write a composite picture of the community to share with their learning group. Each small learning group discusses the exercise and develops a composite picture of the commonalties identified by members of the group. The group consensus summary is posted in a public discussion forum for all groups to read.

4. Good practice gives prompt feedback: technology provides many opportunities for feedback, both synchronous (real time, i.e.,virtual chat), asynchronous (time delayed, i.e., discussion boards) and e-mail. What is considered "prompt" should be clarified in the course directions or in the syllabus. For example, the instructor will post "I will read all posting on the discussion board once a week and will write a comment to the group." "I will answer all e-mails in three working days." "Office hours: I will be available in the virtual chat room on Wednesday from 7 to 8 p.m. Please join me to ask questions or clarify content about computing and interpreting rates."

5. Good practice emphasizes time on task: time is critical and using time wisely is a goal online. Online courses save the student commuting and parking time. Students can learn anywhere, at home or at work, or wherever there is a computer.

A rule of thumb is to double or triple the number of course credits to determine the number of hours a week a student will spend online. For example, a student enrolled in a three-credit course may spend 6 to 9 hours a week in the online course.

6. Good practice communicates high expectations: some students register for online courses because they think it will be easier. Then they find out that is a fallacy. Expectations should be clear with students. If students are not performing at the expected level, the instructor can e-mail the student and describe observed behavior and delineate expected behavior. For example, the instructor sees that a student is posting such comments as "I agree, Cathy" or "great idea, Michelle". The faculty can send an e-mail saying "Mary, I have read your postings and can see that in some you clearly express your ideas and you use the literature to support your ideas and in other postings your comments are less substantiated. I can see that you have excellent ideas and would like to see you share these with your peers."

7. Good practice respects diverse talents and ways of learning: the advantage of online courses is the many resources available to accommodate a variety of learning styles. For example, for the visual learners, use PowerPoint. For the audio learner, use audio-visual material, and for readers, add notes or narrations. Slide shows can be easily constructed for disseminating content online. Links can be added. There can be schedules for students who need structure, for example, each student is expected to post to a discussion at least twice a week.

COLLABORATIVE PARTNERSHIPS

While the guiding principles of quality practice were being developed, universities were struggling with what Noble (1998) calls automation. According to Noble, automation, "the distribution of digitized course material online, without the participation of professors who develop such material—is often justified as an inevitable part of the new knowledge-based society" (Noble, 1998, p. 1). UCLA instituted the "Instructional Enhancement Initiative" which mandated that all arts and science courses have a Web-based delivery component. The university partnered with private corporations and formed its own for-profit company (Noble, 1998). Noble says "it is by no accident that the high-tech transformation of higher education is being initiated and implemented from the top down, either without any student and faculty involvement in the decision-making or despite it" (Noble, 1998, p. 2). Although faculty and students were opposed to the initiative, UCLA administrators continued with their plans (Noble, 1998). Further Noble (1998) cites a reason for the decision to continue—the fear of being left behind in an academic trend. He calls this "the commercialism of higher education (p.3). For here, as elsewhere, technology is but a vehicle and a disarming disguise." The function of the university is to teach and universities are developing their courseware into marketable, sellable products in hopes of getting "a piece of the commercial action for their institutions or themselves, as vendors in their own right of software and content" (Noble, 1998, p. 5). The concern of faculty is the quality of education. Faculty view Web-based instruction as commoditizing education and the fear is that the quality of instruction will be compromised by automation.

Online courses and programs grew from 1999 to 2001 through grants awarded by the Department of Education called Learning Anytime Anywhere Partnerships (LAAP) for innovative distance learning partnerships. Proposed by President Bill Clinton, funds from the Fund for the Improvement of Postsecondary Education reached $10 million in 1999, $23.3 million in 2000, and $30 million in 2001. The project is being phased out (Carnevale, 2001) but the emphasis on partnerships continued to grow.

NURSING ROLES ONLINE

Consumer Health Informatics

Ferguson (1997, p 251) defines consumer health informatics (CHI) as "the study of consumer interfaces in health care systems" and describes two types: community CHI resources and clinical CHI resources. Community resources are those that consumers can access online. Clinical resources are programs or systems that are provided to selected members or patients, i.e. physician-patient e-mail or home health workstations. Ferguson calls health consumers online self-helpers. Online self-helpers go online looking for information, support, and advice. They get this through online support forums that provide information, asynchronous chat, and live chat (Ferguson, 1997). Ferguson (1997) suggests that online self-helpers are able to get:

- answers to questions
- answers to other self-helpers' questions
- information

Ferguson (1997, p. 257) concluded that one of the roots of our current "health care crisis" is our current "professional-as-authority" model of health care. Ferguson cites two laws that will predict the future. First is Moore's Law—that computers will expand exponentially with a resultant increase in bandwidth and decrease in cost. The second law is Metcalf's Law—that the number of computer networks will increase exponentially as the number of people who connect to the network increases. Because of the current trend toward acceptance of online health information, Ferguson (1997) predicts a major transformation will take place that will redefine health care. This prediction is supported by Eysenbach and Diepgen (2001) who describe the convergence of several factors that came together at the same time to promote and expand e-Health. Consumers became more responsible for their own health care at a time when health providers realized the potential of having their consumers gain information and support online. The value of an educated, empowered consumer in improving the quality of health care is recognized. During a time when the cost of health care is an issue, online learning has cost-saving benefits in that consumers can access information and support online. The information age and consumerism have merged to empower consumers and thus improve the quality of health care.

Leaffer and Gonda (2000) titled their journal article "The Internet: An Underutilized Tool in Patient Education." The title summarized their study findings that when senior citizens were taught how to use the internet to search, find, and share health information, 66% continued this behavior in a 90–day follow-up and, 47% continued to search for health information. The seniors who used the Internet to find health information reported more satisfaction with health care as a result of the increased knowledge and discussion with their physician. These findings are relevant to nursing.

Nursing has traditionally played a very strong role in patient education, which now needs to incorporate Internet technology. Nursing curricula needs to be reengineered to incorporate the Internet as a valuable patient education tool in order to prepare both nursing students and nurse practitioners for the healthcare demands of the 21 century. The reengineered curricula will have to consider the significant increase in the number of older patients the nursing profession will have to serve (Leaffer & Gonda, 2000). Nurses should offer seniors the option of using the Internet to search and find health information. Nursing faculty should use the Internet to access health information in nursing curricula, and student nurses should be taught how to use the Internet as a source of health information and how to teach clients to use the Internet effectively to obtain information.

Continuing Education and Training

In a 1998 article Plank writes "if the Internet is not recognized and used for educational purposes by nurses, those nurses will be left behind" (p. 166). The Internet offers "a unique opportunity to provide innovative approaches to career mobility for registered nurses" (O'Brien & Renner, 2000, p.13) because the Internet provides a cost-effective and accessible method of imparting information to nurses. The challenges are that the nurses need to have (or learn) technical skills and communication skills to interact online.

Mandatory continuing education offers a unique opportunity to nurses for online continuing education as an alternative to the classroom. The advantages (Bergren, 1999) for School Nurses are that they can learn at their own pace and on their own schedule, and can learn about topics of importance and interest to them. Cobb & Baird (1999) reported on the use of the Internet for continuing education for oncology nurses. The nurses ask for oncology related news, chat for symptom management, legislative news, bulletin boards, and legislative e-mails.

The Internet is an option for certification review courses. Family or Adult Nurse Practitioner Certification Examination review courses online offer the nurse guidance and support through interactive learning, audiovisual presentations, exercises, practice tests, and links to resources (Web Options, 2000).

Nursing Students

The American Association of Colleges of Nursing (AACN) approved a white paper, Distance Technology in Nursing Education developed by the AACN Task Force on Distance Technology and Nursing Education on July 26, 1999. The importance of technology in nursing education is recognized. The focus of the white paper is using technology to enhance nursing education. To do so, schools must strategically plan for distance education programs. Several factors need to be addressed by nursing and other leaders in education and health care institutions, as well as by external funders and policy makers:

- Superior distance education programs require substantial institutional financial investment in equipment, infrastructure, and faculty development.
- Local, regional, and national planning for multisite communications need to consider coordination of services, compatibility and progressive upgrading of hardware, as well as policies that lower transmission costs within and across state lines.
- The use of distance technology and, in particular, Web-based media, has raised questions regarding intellectual property and copyrights, privacy of educational dialogue, and other related legal and ethical issues that require continued clarification.
- Technology-mediated teaching strategies can dramatically

change the way teaching and learning occurs, challenging the traditional relationship of students to academic institutions. These strategies may change conventional thinking about how quality of educational programs is assessed and what is required to support student learning (e.g., library access, counseling services, computing equipment, tuition, and financial aid).

- Distance education technology has provided some nursing schools an advantage in recruiting students and is increasing competition among institutions (AACN, July, 1999).

The AACN (January, 2000) outlines differences in distance education from traditional learning in nursing. In distance education student and faculty roles change. The teacher moves from sage-on-the-stage to guide-on-the-side, and students interact more and become more cohesive. Distance learning is a strategy that will boost enrollment in schools of nursing (AACN June, 2000; January, 2000) because it will attract students who would not enroll in traditional programs. Distance education gives faculty an opportunity to use technology to teach in new and creative ways. Distance education can open the doors to more collaboration through partnerships to share resources and faculty expertise.

SUMMARY

Whether the nurse is developing an intranet site, orienting new nurses, updating skills for nurses, teaching consumers, teaching student nurses, or developing continuing education programs in online environments, a basic set of skills are necessary. Those skills include:

- Having an understanding of the impact of infrastructure, resources, and supports in imparting information and communicating online
- Understanding pedagogy in order to make decisions about what to teach and how to effectively teach it
- Having knowledge and skills in technology to be able to develop Web sites and put information online

- Reconceptualizing learning to online environments
- Using pedagogy and technology to design creative, effective learning environments online
- Teaching and communicating in online environments
- Assessing and evaluating learning online

With basic knowledge and understanding of these skills the nurse can begin to effectively build quality online learning environments for teaching students. In addition, with these skills, the nurse can develop learning environments for consumers and professional peers.

REFERENCES

American Association of Colleges of Nursing (January 2000). *Distance learning is changing and challenging nursing education.* Retrieved July 18, 2002, from *http://aacn.nche.edu/Publications/issues/jan2000.htm.*

American Association of Colleges of Nursing (July 1999). *AACN white paper: Distance technology in nursing education.* Retrieved July 18, 2002, from *http://aacn.nche.edu?Publications/positions/whitepaper.htm.*

American Association of Colleges of Nursing (June 2000). *Amid nursing shortages, schools employ strategies to boost enrollment.* Retrieved July 11, 2002, from *http://www.aacn.nche.edu/Publications/issues/ib600wb.htm*

American Council on Education (n.d.). *Center for adult learning.* Retrieved July 10, 2002, from *http://www.acenet.edu/calec/dist_learning/dl_definitions.cfm*

Bergren, M.D. (1999). Online continuing education. *Journal of School Nursing.* 15(4), 32–34.

Carnevale, D. (September 28, 2001). Education Department cuts new distance-education grants. *The Chronicle of Higher Education.* Retrieved July 17, 2002 from *http://chronicle.com*

Chickering, A.W. & Ehrmann, S.C. (1996). *AAHE Bulletin, October.* Retrieved June 23, 2002, from *http://www.tltgroup.org/programs/seven.html.*

Cobb, S.C. & Baird, S.B. (1999). Oncology nurses' use of the internet for continuing education: A survey of oncology nursing society congress attendees. *The Journal of Continuing Education in Nursing.* 30(5), 199–202.

Eysenbach, G. & Diepgen, T. (2001). The role of e-health and consumer health informatics for evidence-based patient choice in the 21st century. *Clinics in Dermatology,* 19, 11–17.

Ferguson, T. (1997). Health online and the empowered medical consumer. *Journal on Quality Improvement*, 23(5), 251–257.

Khan, B.H. (1997). *Web-based instruction*. Englewood Cliffts, NJ: Educational Technology Publications, Inc.

Leaffer, T. & Gonda, B. (2000). The Internet: An underutilized tool in patient education. *Computers in Nursing*, 18(1), 47–52.

Merisotis, J.P. & Phipps, R.A. (1999). What's the difference? A review of contemporary research on the effectiveness of distance learning in higher education. Washington D.C.; The Institute for Higher Education Policy.

Noble, D.F. (1998). *Digital diploma mills: The automation of higher education*. Retrieved July 21, 2002, from *http://www.firstmonday.dk/issues/issue3_1/noble*.

O'Brien, B.S. & Renner, A. (2000). Nurses online: Career mobility for registered nurses. *Journal of Professional Nursing*, 16(1), pp. 13–20.

Plank, K.P. (1998). Nursing on-line for continuing education credit. *The Journal of Continuing Education in Nursing*. 29(4), pp. 165–172.

Russell, T. (1998). *No significant difference: Phenomenon as reported in 248 research reports, summaries, and papers* (4th ed.). Raleigh: North Carolina State University.

Web Options. (2000). "*What's New*", 26(4), 41A.

Young, J.F. (March 22, 2002). "Hybrid" teaching seeks to end the divide between traditional and online instruction. *The Chronicle of Higher Education*. Retrieved July 17, 2002 from *http://chronicle.com*.

2

Theories of Learning and the Online Environment

Technology has allowed for a broader reach to students and thus has expanded access to education. Expanding access in nursing is important for two reasons: the nursing shortage and the emphasis on increasing the number of BSN nurses. Potential nursing students may be employed full time, have families, and not have the time to attend traditional educational programs. By providing online learning environments and thereby enhancing access, more students may enroll in nursing educational programs and thus reduce the nursing shortage. To meet the complex demands of today's health care environment, a federal advisory panel has recommended that at least two-thirds of the basic nurse workforce hold baccalaureate or higher degrees in nursing by 2010. Aware of this need, RNs are seeking the BSN degree in increasing numbers (American Association of Colleges of Nursing, 2000). To meet increased demand for online learning opportunities, partnerships among universities have developed to allow for sharing of resources and to enhance the quality of online learning in both national and international perspectives.

ONLINE AND FACE-TO-FACE LEARNING ENVIRONMENTS

What are the differences between online and face-to-face learning environments? Online learning is accessible anytime and anywhere which makes it convenient for the learner. One reason is because online learning is only technology dependent. If the technology is available, so is the learning. Face-to-face learning is scheduled and classes are offered at set times in specific places. The course a learner needs may be offered 50 miles away at 8 a.m. The student must be available when and where the course is offered. Face-to-face learning tends to be a one-size-fits-all approach, some with large classes, and with lecture as the major teaching modality.

In online learning environments, students can log on and review their course material whenever they want and wherever a computer with Internet access is available. Online students are spared driving to class during winter months in snow-prone locations. They are also spared the inconvenience of traffic, the unavailability and cost of parking, and compromised safety, especially in cities with night classes.

Since learning online is technology dependent, the GIGO rule applies: Garbage In—Garbage Out. Online learning is not "slapping classroom content online". Online learning is using the positive resources of technology to bring learning content and experiences to learners. In other words, use the resource to enhance the content. Dr. Drucker (2000, p. 5) of the Delphi Group wrote in a white paper on e-learning that "the power of e-learning rests in its ability to deliver both the richness and reach needed to maximize the effectiveness of the learning process". Learning online is thought to be a lonely and isolated experience because online learners cannot see each other and the teacher cannot see the students. If you can't see them, you can't teach them, seems to be a traditionalist mantra. Going back to GIGO, online learning that excludes interaction denies the learner of a quality learning experience. Online learners should be actively interacting with each other (student to student) and with teachers (student to teacher).

Dr. Drucker (2000, p.5) calls online learning high in personalization to the user and the task. "By providing the tools by which a user can fully personalize the experience based on their skills and tasks, e-learning creates a much more intimate and memorable (i.e., effective) learning experience." Dr. Drucker (2000) describes e-learning as having just-in-time and personalized content, and academic education as having just-in-case and generalized content.

Khan (1997) describes the key features of Web-based instruction: interactivity and design mediums that take advantage of multimedia available on the Web. Other key features are:

- Online search/resources and electronic publishing
- Uniformity worldwide enabling nondiscriminatory, cross-cultural interaction
- Industry supported
- Learner-controlled, convenient, self contained, easy to use, friendly, and cost effective
- Course is secure
- Collaborative learning

Cravener (1999) delineates the differences between traditional and Web-based instruction in regards to faculty workload, accessing education, adapting to technology, and instructional quality. She writes that online courses are more time consuming and labor intensive. There is increased access to instruction and other educational resources. There is an imperative need to teach students to use the technology. There is a lack of visual and nonvisual cues in online interactions. Online production teams are needed to develop and implement courses. More planning and preparation of instructional material and contingency plans are needed online. Online courses need to be highly organized which may result in the loss of improvisation. There is the potential for increased collaborative learning activities online. More faculty-student interaction opportunities are available online. Cravener also outlines three advantages of web-based instruction: increased access, improved quality and reduced cost. She says having all three is not realistic. So, pick two.

CHARACTERISTICS OF ONLINE COURSES

Online learning experiences consist of: an audience, a purpose, learning objectives, content, multimedia design, interaction (synchronous and asynchronous), and assessment and evaluation activities. In an online learning module, there are objectives that tell the learner what they will accomplish and they guide the design. In addition, orientation and support services are provided for teachers and learners. A learning module should be about 50% self study and 50% interaction. The format for the learner is to read the material, do the assignments (activity), discuss the assignments, and then report on the assignment. Drucker (2000, p. 5) describes the power of e-learning as its ability to deliver richness to the learning process.

> Richness in presentation is provided by multimedia technologies, allowing both a live classroom experience, as well as synchronous modes which include audio and video. Content richness is provided by blending off-the-shelf learning materials with custom materials and internal knowledge. Equally important, richness is provided by integrating content in context, making it timely and relevant to business operations.

Illinois Online Network (ION) cites the key elements of an online program as the students, the curriculum, the facilitator, and the technology. Students must have a positive attitude, skills, and commitment to be a good candidate for online learning. Courses should be organized and should focus on applying what is learned to the real world and foster critical thinking and the exchange of ideas with students and faculty.

> Online curriculum has two important aspects, process and outcomes. The process must integrate life, work and educational experience, include ample time for the completion of the assigned work, utilize a minimal amount of memorization, maintain a balance between the technology, the facilitator and the students, and incorporate group and team activities. The learning outcomes must be achievable and offer the opportunity for students to use them in practical, everyday situations. (ION, 2002)
>
> The facilitator is responsible for the appropriate design of the curriculum and facilitation of the course. Technology is a tool for learning and it should be user friendly, reliable, accessible and affordable. The technology should accommodate the lowest common denominator of the class.

THEORIES IN EDUCATION

Theories about learning are mostly derived from psychology. While psychology describes how people act, educational theory describes how people learn. We can use educational theories therefore to design and implement effective educational programs.

Behaviorism was one of the most influential theories in the education and psychology field. Ivan Pavlov (1849–1936) conducted experiments in Russia with dogs. He rang a bell and then gave the dogs food. He repeated the ringing of the bell and the giving of food over and over until the dogs began to salivate in anticipation of food when the bell rang. This stimulus-response behavior is called classic conditioning. Edward Thorndike (1874–1949) applied behaviorism to education at Columbia University in New York. He postulated that learning was the resultant connection between a stimulus and a response. John B. Watson, who is often referred to as the true father of behaviorism, earned his Ph.D. at the University of Chicago in 1903. Watson's research connected conditioned fear and emotional response.

B.F. Skinner (1904–1990) continued work with stimulus-response but focused on studying voluntary responses. He rewarded responses that were desirable and punished or ignored undesirable responses. His work is called operant conditioning. His theory, like those of Pavlov, Thorndike and Watson, were based on behavioral change while mental processes were ignored. Behavioral change is what is observed, for example, what one is saying, or does, or how one behaves. If a behavior is observed, it is the response to a stimulus. A stimulus is defined as an object in the environment that poses a physiologic threat. A response is anything that one does in response to a stimulus. It could be as simple as a turn of the head, a twitch, or saying, "I am sorry," or as complex as designing a building or writing a book. Behaviorism was popular into the 1940s and 1950s but began to lose supporters because the theory explained learning from only a behavioral perspective and is therefore limited in scope.

The psychological theory of behaviorism is used as an educational theory when the learning experience is based on a stimulus and a response and by rewarding behavior that will meet the educational goal and ignoring (or correcting) behavior that is not goal directed.

In behavioral theory, large tasks are broken down into smaller tasks, and each task is learned in successive order. The process is called successive approximations. Traditional learning labs are an example of behaviorist theory and one nursing example is learning the correct procedure for a dry, sterile dressing. By taking the entire procedure and breaking it down into steps, the learner masters the first step then moves to the next step and so on until he/she masters every step to complete the procedure. The first step would be to verify the order, then gather equipment, then prepare the client, then set up the area for a sterile field, etc. By learning a segment at a time and doing each segment correctly, the student will be able to successfully complete the dry sterile dressing procedure by putting the learned steps together.

Bandura suggested a Social Cognitive Theory of learning in which information is stored in schema. When new information is internalized, it is compared with existing information. Schemas reorganize to accommodate the new information. Sensory input is stored for several seconds. If it is deemed unimportant, it disappears. If it is important, it is transferred to short-term memory for a period of time. If it continues to be important, it is moved to long-term memory. Long-term memory has unlimited capacity and storage space. In this theory, new information is linked to existing information and therefore thought patterns are changed.

In nursing we may be teaching a woman to perform monthly breast self-examinations. We first assess the woman's knowledge about doing exams. Then we would give her pamphlets with instructions and show a video. We might show the woman the procedure for performing an effective exam. We give the woman information and in social cognitive theory it is assumed that this new information is added to existing information and therefore the woman will learn how to accurately perform a breast self-assessment.

Cognitive theory is used in the traditional classroom to impart information from the teacher to the student. The teacher lectures, uses Power Point, films, guest speakers, panel discussions, and many other methods of imparting information. The responsibility for learning lies with the student. The student is expected to take in the new knowledge and the assumption is that if the student takes knowledge in, it will be transformed into new thought processes. The weakness of cognitivism is its inability to explain human thought and learning.

CONSTRUCTIVISM THEORY

Some educators believe that the teacher can impart information but that does not mean that the student will learn. These educators believe that learning occurs when the learner uses information to think. Thinking inspires learning. Thinking is stimulated through activities. It is the teacher who provides the content and the activities and initiates and motivates the learner to involve themselves in the activities and thus to think. Thinking helps the learner to transform information to their context or a context personal to them and thus see ways to use the information in their lives. Learning becomes the responsibility of the learner.

Jonassen, Peck, Wilson and Pfeiffer (1998) contrast traditional learning and constructivism. In traditional learning, knowledge is transmitted and is external to the learner, whereas in constructivist learning knowledge is constructed by the learner's action, experience, and perceptions. In traditional learning methods learning is the transfer of knowledge from the teacher to the student with an emphasis on the outcome. Constructivist learning focuses on interpreting the world and in constructing meaning. Learning is active and reflective which means that there is doing, then reflecting about the doing and then rethinking about the doing. Action and reflection enables the student to integrate new knowledge with existing knowledge and experiences so that complex mental models can form. Integrating the old and the new learning allows the student to look at the world from a unique perspective. Learning is authentic and resembles real-life experiences. Constructivist learning is process oriented with an emphasis on collaboration and conversation among learners and teachers. Instruction also differs. In the traditional classroom instruction is the imparting of information from the top, down using a deductive thinking process. Learning is competitive and is controlled by the instructor. In the constructivist approach instruction is inductive and from the bottom, up. Learning opportunities are diverse and increase in complexity. The instructor is a model and a coach who encourages exploration of ideas, and learning is learner-centered and learner-generated.

Constructivism assumes that learning is personal and that the student brings past knowledge and experience to the learning situation. Constructivism is the process of bringing new knowledge to past experiences to construct a new reality and make sense and meaning out of the world. How do students construct their own reality? It is through engaging in an active learning process. Active learning is an approach that engages the student in thinking and rethinking, thus creating new ideas. Students interact with the environment (content, faculty, activities, peers). Active learning according to Dodge (no date) involves the process of providing students with situations which require them to read, speak, listen, think, and write. Although lectures may be well-written and well-delivered, they often pass from the ear to the hand leaving the mind untouched. The active learning process places responsibility on the learners themselves and lends itself to a wider range of learning styles. Active learning on the Web involves a critical look at the resources that already exist and incorporating them into the learning environment. Examples might include Web quests or newsgroups that would require learners to research information then return to the online class environment to further collaborate and expand on their research findings.

If the student constructs meaning from content, faculty, activities, and peers, then learning environments must be rich with strategies and resources. Technology can provide the richness constructivist learning environments need to guide knowledge construction.

TECHNOLOGY AND LEARNING

Technology has traditionally been used for the purpose of conveying information to students. Jonassen, Peck, Wilson and Pfeiffer

(1998) suggest that technology does more—that technology can be used to support the student creating meaning out of learning. Technology can foster learning because:

- Technology is a tool that can be used to support knowledge construction. Technology allows students to share knowledge and experience and build mental models.
- Technology is an information vehicle for exploring knowledge to support learning-by-constructing. Technology allows access to information and databases in the acquision of knowledge.
- Technology supports learning by doing. Technology supports simulations and case studies that are real-world problems. Technology provides an opportunity for students to solve these problems in a safe, supportive environment.
- Technology is a social medium that supports student learning by conversing. Through synchronous and asynchronous learning, students can discuss and build consensus.
- Technology is an intellectual partner that supports learning by reflecting. Technology can provide learners with ways to articulate and represent what they know.

So, how can we bring learning theory and technology together to create effective learning environments? Undergraduate nursing education traditionally includes faculty/teacher developed behavioral objectives, with content developed by faculty/teacher to meet the objectives and evaluation that focuses on the attainment of objectives. This faculty/teacher-centered approach is an example of behaviorism. The teacher is responsible for focusing on:

- Identification of relevant stimuli and response
- Identification of the learner's entry level and the setting of student expectations
- Analysis of learner skills and knowledge
- Planning a reinforcement schedule
- Constant confirmation of expectations; maintenance of motivation
- Development of individualized instruction and seatwork exercises

- Constant assessment of learning each skill before progressing to another skill

The student's role is to achieve the objectives. Nursing uses objectives to guide and evaluate learning, and objectives are an integral component of nursing education and training. Here is the dilemma: Behaviorism is teacher centered and online learning should be student centered. Nursing education/training tends toward behaviorism, and the literature supports constructivism as the online approach to effective learning. If teacher-centered objectives and outcome measures of evaluation are a necessity, techniques can be used to make the behaviorist favor constructivist components and thereby become more student centered. One technique is to include assessments of student learning styles and structure learning experiences to accommodate those learning styles. Once learning style is assessed, develop a prescriptive plan for each student to guide their learning. Objectives can be written in a behavioral format, but students can provide real-life case studies to analyze and thus meet objectives. When a combination of behaviorist and constructivist approaches are used, the learning is called a "guided constructivist learning model".

If guided constructivism were the theory used to design online learning environments, objectives would be teacher centered and would guide the learning experience. An emphasis would be placed on the process of knowledge construction rather than on the outcomes of learning. Content would be presented to accommodate various learning styles and an emphasis would be placed on active learning through questions, case studies, and projects that would help the student develop mental models and test reality. These approaches would allow the student to apply basic information to real world practice.

SUCCESSFUL ONLINE STUDENTS

Successful online students have common characteristics. Such as:

- Highly motivated, independent, and active learners.
- Good organizational and time management skills.

- Disciplined to study without external reminders.
- Adaptable to new learning environments.

Illinois Online Network (undated) suggests that the students who most benefit from online learning are homebound, live long distances from the campus and have busy lives with families, a profession, and other responsibilities. The successful student is mature, open-minded, self-motivated, accepting of critical thinking, willing to work collaboratively, has good written communication skills, and has a minimum level of technological experience.

What are the providers of online learning telling their potential students about what makes a successful online student? Included in the online resource material for Illinois Online Network, is a list of qualities that include:

- Be open minded about sharing life, work, and educational experiences as part of the learning process.
- Be able to communicate through writing and be willing to "speak up" if problems arise.
- Be self-motivated and self-disciplined and willing and able to commit to 4 to 15 hours per week per course.
- Accept critical thinking and decision making as part of the learning process.
- Have access to a computer and a modem.
- Be able to think ideas through before responding.
- Feel that high quality learning can take place without going to a traditional classroom.

The Collaborative Nursing Program (undated) is an online baccalaureate degree program for registered nurses that was started in 1996 and is offered by the University of Wisconsin (UW) Eau Claire, Green Bay, Madison, Milwaukee and Oshkosh campuses. This program targets underserved RNs in remote, rural areas. The student orientation guidelines include study strategy tips for success:

- Advanced organization and preparation: arrange for time to study.

- Develop a study plan.
- Create a study environment.
- Work alone and with study partners.
- Apply what you are learning.
- Speak up.

This site also offers advice from experienced distance learners to inexperienced distance learners:

- Be committed (4 to 15 hours per week per course) and take the program and yourself seriously.
- Prioritize because as you will need to make choices.
- Have private study space and find a buddy.
- Be self-motivated and self-disciplined and take responsibility for your own learning.
- Participate, be active and involved, log on every day, and keep up with the class.
- Use online conferencing.
- Communicate in writing.
- Be open-minded, think critically, and speak up.
- Apply what you learn.
- Use proper "netiquette."

The HTML Writers Guild (undated) was founded in 1994 as an educational organization for web developers. They offer Guidelines for a Successful Online Class Experience that includes the following.

- Order your book early.
- Have any required software installed before class begins.
- Be sure you have the correct software.
- Be sure you meet any skills prerequisites.
- Late registration requires immediate access to texts and software.
- Plan your studies wisely.
- Access your classroom several times a week.
- Keep all e-mail regarding your courses.
- Enjoy yourself.

SUMMARY

Learning in online environments is an educational methodology that is most effective when based on constructivist learning theory. Nursing uses behavioral objectives to guide learning. Online learning in nursing can use a constructivist approach but must also include behaviorism; thus the term guided constructivism is used to describe teaching and learning nursing online. The successful online student: organizes learning time and space, schedules time to study, interacts and communicates and keeps up with the rest of the class.

REFERENCES

American Association of College of Nursing (2000). *Strategies to reverse the new nursing shortage.* Retrieved June 23, 2002, from *http://www.aacn.nche.edu/Media/Backgrounders/nursfact.htm.*

Cravener, P.A. (1999). *Faculty experiences with providing online courses: Thorns among the roses.* Computers in Nursing, 17(1), 42–47.

Dodge, B. (no date). *Active learning on the web.* Retrieved June 24, 2002, from *http://edweb.sdsu.edu/people/bdodge/Active/ActiveLearning.html.*

Drucker, P. (2000). *Need to know: Integrating e-Learning with high velocity value chains.* Boston: Delphi Group.

Graham, G. (2002). *Stanford encyclopedia of philosophy.* Retrieved June 24, 2002, from *http://plato.stanford.edu/entries/behaviorism/#1.*

Jonassen, D.H., Peck, K.L., Wilson, B.G. & Pfeiffer, W.S. (1998). *Learning with technology: A constructivist perspective.* New Jersey: Prentice Hall.

Illinois Online Network (ION). Retrieved June 24, 2002, from *http://illinois.online.uillinois.edu.*

Khan, B. (1997). *Web-Based Instruction.* New Jersey: Educational Technology Publications.

The Collaborative Nursing Program. Retrieved June 24, 2002, from *http://www.uwex.edu/disted/cnp.*

The HTML Writers Guild. Retrieved June 24, 2002, from *http://www.hwg.org.*

Western Cooperative for Educational Telecommunications. Retrieved on June 29, 2002 from *http://www.wiche.edu.*

3

Developing the Infrastructure for Online Learning: Student, Faculty, and Technical Support

Infrastructure is a conglomeration of policies, services, technology, and resources designated to support distance-learning efforts. A distance-learning program needs an efficient and effective infrastructure to be successful. Building infrastructure is dependent on institutional issues, technological issues, student support services, and faculty support. Berge and Schrum (1998) propose that there is a need to conduct planning and programmatic implementation simultaneously, and to integrate these activities into the fabric of the institution as seamlessly as possible. This may or may not be a reality for most institutions. In many cases, institutions are attempting to operate an online program based on existing resources and policies. This chapter will address major factors and issues that need consideration when planning a distance education program within the broad scope of the supporting infrastructure elements.

A good place to start is by looking at the institution's mission and strategic plan for evidence of support of online learning. Pennsylvania State University, a longstanding leader in distance education, developed guiding principles for infrastructure to support distance education and they are based on policy, a dynamic programmatic mission, student and faculty support and the need for policy change to support distance education efforts. Pennsylvania State University maintains that distance education is best recognized as an integrated part of the college-wide strategic goals and not as a separate activity. Distance courses allow for global reach and expansion of an academic setting by increasing the availability of courses.

The American Association of Colleges of Nursing (AACN) (1999) identifies factors that need to be addressed by nursing and other leaders in education and health care institutions, as well as external funders and policy makers, in order to take full advantage of the benefits of technology supported education. These factors include:

- Superior distance education programs require substantial institutional financial investment in equipment, infrastructure, and faculty development.
- Local, regional, and national planning for multisite communications needs to consider coordination of services, compatibility and progressive upgrading of hardware, as well as policies that lower transmission costs within and across state lines.
- The use of distance technology and Web-based media in particular, has raised questions regarding intellectual property and copyrights, privacy of educational dialogue, and other related legal and ethical issues that require continued clarification.
- Technology-mediated teaching strategies can dramatically change the way teaching and learning occurs, challenging the traditional relationship of students to academic institutions. These strategies may change conventional thinking about how quality of educational programs is assessed and what is required to support student learning (e.g., library access, counseling services, computing equipment, tuition, and financial aid).
- Nursing schools that use distance education technology have an advantage in recruiting students and nursing schools are competing for students in their distance programs.

With knowledge of the supporting documents and elements that need to be in place, an institution can better assess and plan where to focus resources and efforts necessary for a successful online program infrastructure.

INSTITUTIONAL SUPPORT

The mission statement and strategic plan are important documents to begin to develop or analyze infrastructure because it is within these documents that the future direction and long range plans can be identified in terms of both human and technological support for distance learning. The American Distance Education Consortium (ADEC) (2002) has developed guiding principles for distance learning and discusses key issues such as developing and maintaining technological and human infrastructure issues related to administrative and organizational commitment. The institution should be supportive of the needs of the learners. The ADEC recommends that all opportunities for distance students be disclosed. Tutorial support, registration, advising, counseling, library and other information services, and problem solving assistance would be some of these support services.

The National Academic Advising Association (NACADA) (1999) developed the following institutional standards:

- Provide leadership and an organizational structure that integrates and coordinates activities that support distance learning for faculty, advisors, and students.
- Truth in advertising: Recruitment and admissions promotions must accurately represent the program and available services.
- Be committed to the concept of distance education by providing ongoing technical and financial support for a period sufficient to enable students to complete a degree or certificate.
- The institution has an obligation to work toward providing the same student services to distance learners as they do for students on campus.
- The institutional philosophy concerning the distance learning support services program must be to strive to respond to learner needs rather than the learner adjusting to an institution's established organizational structure.
- Continuous evaluation is an institutional responsibility to determine the program's educational effectiveness, assess

student learning outcomes, analyze student retention, and measure the level of student/ faculty satisfaction.
- Institute an orientation course, i.e., DL 101 "What it takes to be a successful distance learner."
- Proper assessment must be conducted to ensure students have the required backgrounds, knowledge, and technical skills needed to undertake the program.

The University of Hawaii's Community College's distance learning strategic plan states that "each campus strives to meet its community's needs and distance education has been one of the means utilized". Building on years of experience, the UHCC system has made a commitment to collaboratively deliver degrees via distance technologies. This commitment, in effect, became a logical step once the UH system made a decision to use distance learning to improve access within its communities.

Virginia Tech's strategic plan for distance learning states that "its most explicit goal is to strengthen Virginia Tech's role as a recognized leader in distance and distributed teaching and learning, research and scholarship, outreach and public service." Distance and distributed learning is an integral part of the university's academic agenda and is part of this university's effort to be recognized as one of the top universities in the country. The statements by all these universities demonstrate the commitment of their efforts and resources to their distance programs.

INFORMATION TECHNOLOGY

A significant technological infrastructure will be necessary to deliver a serious and comprehensive distance-learning program. This infrastructure might include studios, large servers, support and help desks, and a high-speed high capacity network (Hawkins, 1999). Currently many campuses are considering whether they are positioned to provide the requisite technological investment and what their role might be in a distributed or distance education arena. Collaboration, consortia and other alliances could allow campuses to contribute content and resources to specific courses or areas of study in order to make most efficient use of time and money. "Content that can't be deployed over the network because of bandwidth or connectivity problems is useless," advises Kelly. "Understand the IT standards, and then innovate around those standards and practices" (Delahoussaye, Zemke, & Miller, 2001. p3).

When addressing technological and human infrastructure issues, the ADEC recommends that appropriate technical requirements be established, compatibility needs be met, technology at origination and reception sites assure quality, learners and facilitators be supported in their use of these technologies, and collaboration efforts be explored. It is becoming increasingly common to find institutional settings seeking external collaboration opportunities in order to share resources.

The Western Interstate Commission for Higher Education (WICHE) was established by the western states to promote resource sharing, collaboration, and cooperative planning among their higher education systems. These systems share program resources, information and technical expertise, services, and equipment related to distance learning. Wireless computing is predicted to be more powerful and pervasive in the future and will have implications for higher education. Information security and privacy of information have always been of concern and will need to be addressed to ensure the protection of student data.

The development of statewide telecommunications efforts is underway in Indiana to deliver data, video and voice on the concept of partnership and collaboration. The primary advantage is the overall level of involvement in the direction and policy development guiding the network. Similarly, the Iowa Communication Network (ICN) invests in educational telecommunications and technology to support two-way interactive video conferencing. The network uses T-1 connections, or better for Internet access and long-distance telephone service. The use of the ICN for distance learning is supported by state funds so the cost for schools to use the distance-learning network is very affordable.

STUDENT SUPPORT SERVICES

The Western Cooperative for Telecommunications Education (1999) developed a guide for developing distance student services. These guidelines discuss tips for developing these services in addition to a discussion on the range of services that should be included and guidelines for best practices in delivering these services online. Although universities have increasingly recognized the value and need to provide online courses and programs, they often need help envisioning what services to provide and how to design them. The services addressed in this guide for students were determined to be "good practices" based on interactive web services or for-profit companies that market software to support student needs. The student support services identified include:

- Information for prospective students
- Admissions
- Financial aid
- Registration
- Orientation services
- Academic advising
- Technical support
- Career services
- Library services
- Services for students with disabilities
- Personal counseling
- Instructional support and counseling
- Bookstore
- Services to promote a sense of community

INFORMATION FOR PROSPECTIVE STUDENTS

The services recommended in these guidelines begin with the first encounter that students are likely to have with a university when looking for an online courses or program. The university home page should include information for students to help them decide if this is the right place for them. Recommendations for information include clear and highly visible information about online programs with direct links to more in-depth information. A personal readiness assessment (Example *http://wwww.wqu.edu/wqu/self.assessment.asp)* is recommended to help the student determine if they are ready for online learning. Although these tools do not provide assurance of success, they help students identify technical skills and learning styles that will help them be successful online learners. A hardware and software assessment should be provided to students so they can determine the specifications necessary to participate in a course. A list of hardware, software, Internet Service Provider, e-mail and browser requirements should be specified with definitions of terms included. A FAQ is also often helpful along with contact information such as e-mail or phone numbers for students to get additional information.

ADMISSIONS

The admissions process should be clearly delineated with specific steps for each part of the process. Admission requirements should be identified and program specific criteria would help students decide if they, in fact, want to apply. Methods for obtaining and submitting an application, deadlines, application tracking, and multiple payment methods are also recommended.

Another early step in the process that students should consider is a computer self-assessment. Many universities offering online education have these assessments available on the home page of their Web site. These assessments usually cover basic skills in Windows®, e-mail, hardware, and software. An example of such an assessment can be found at: http://www.units.muohio.edu/mcs/suppctr/lis/Web-Forms/ProfSelfAssessment.shtml

FINANCIAL AID

Financial aid, according to the Western Cooperative, is a critical factor for students in the educational choices that they make. The issue of financial aid has an impact on course load, institutional choice, and whether or not the student can pursue higher education. Because of its importance, students should be able to easily access all financial aid information from the Web. The information should include general information about financial aid, types of aid, details of cost, and the application process. The institutional financial aid policies should be disclosed for students in addition to federal school codes for the federal financial aid application. Dates, deadlines for application, and links to related sites are also important information sources and include general information for students.

Legislation supporting distance students and distance programs can be observed by the recent passing of the Internet Equity and Education Act of 2001 (HR 1992). This bill will modify the "50 % rule" which allows institutions to offer more than 50 % of their class by telecommunications if the institution already participates in the student loan programs and if the institution's, student loan default rate is less than 10 % for the three most recent years. The bill also eliminates the burdensome "12–hour rule" applicable to nonstandard term programs and instead requires that term programs that are offered on a nonsemester basis be held to the same attendance criteria as those offered on a traditional semester basis. Additionally this bill requires that institutions participating in federal financial aid programs submit annual reports on subjects such as types of students participating in distance education, the amount of federal aid used and claims of violations of the Act. Originally the logic behind both the 50% rule and the 12–hour rule was to maintain integrity of the instructional programs being offered to students receiving financial aid. In 1992, the Higher Education Act amendments excluded schools that offered more than half of their courses by correspondence, which included distance education courses. The 12–hour rule was a result of an instructional time mandate. With new instructional delivery modes offered by new technologies, there are now many ways of engaging fully in education that do not involve sitting in a classroom. Opponents to the bill claim that no one has yet come up with an acceptable way to measure equivalency of effort and accomplishments across institutions and disciplines. Thus the U.S. congress has compromised by requiring annual reports of violations.

REGISTRATION

Registration for online students is probably one of the most important online services that must be available and user friendly. This service will be used when students are registering for a program and each time they register for a course. Good practice recommendations include a full description of the registration process, identification of all registration method options available, relevant policies, an online scheduler, and online registration forms with clear instructions. It is important to note that many institutions have developed highly effective touch tone registration systems, which may also serve distance student's needs.

Software for online student registration is increasing in its availability, and ease of use, with increasing ability to meet student and higher education demands. Peoplesoft and Aceware Systems, for example, provide features such as student registration, data-based course management, credit card payment capability, and custom report writing just to mention a few. Additional features include financial aid application capability, records and registration, and the billing system. The Banner system is another popular software, described as a suite of products designed to meet the needs of higher educational institutions. This software manages institutional resources, student information, financial information, and human resources, among others. Various components can be used for faculty, students, advisors and Banner Web employees. This system has the ability to be accessed from home, class, or kiosk in response to calls for flexibility of support services.

LIBRARY SERVICES

Within this constellation of support services, the library is also considered one of the most important. The librarians, library services, and the support staff are all going to be impacted by distance students. No longer will "normal library hours" apply. It will now be necessary to have a Digital Librarian and other specialized staff well versed in managing large databases and electronic resources. The Association of College and Research Libraries (ACRL) (2002) "Guidelines for Distance Learning Library Services" calls for a librarian-administrator to plan, implement, coordinate, and evaluate library resources and services to address the information and skill needs of distance students. The guidelines further state in this document that traditional on-campus library services themselves cannot be stretched to meet the library needs of distance learning students and faculty who face distinct and different challenges involving library access and information delivery. Special funding, proactive planning, and promotion are necessary to deliver equivalent library services to achieve equivalent results in teaching and learning, and generally to maintain quality in distance learning programs. Library services mentioned by the ACLR include:

1. Reference assistance
2. Computer-based bibliographic and informational services
3. Reliable, rapid, secure access to institutional and other networks including the Internet
4. A program of library user instruction designed to instill independent and effective information literacy skills while specifically meeting the learner-support needs of the distance learning community
5. Assistance with and instruction in the use of nonprint media and equipment
6. Reciprocal or contractual borrowing, or interlibrary loan services using broadest application of fair use of copyrighted materials
7. Prompt document delivery such as a courier system and/or electronic transmission
8. Access to reserve materials in accordance with copyright fair use policies
9. Adequate service hours for optimum access by users and consultative services
10. Promotion of library services to the distance learning community, including documented and updated policies, regulations, and procedures for systematic development and management of information resources.

As demand for delivery of these services electronically increases, demand for additional texts, journals, and other resources will also increase.

STUDENT SERVICES

Counseling services need to be available to distance students and can be provided via synchronous or asynchronous means (chat room or e-mail) or by telephone. Student counseling centers often educate through informational pamphlets on various topics. The commercially available options are limited to specialized topics relevant to students. A counseling center can produce its own pamphlets, however, that would otherwise be costly and time consuming. An innovative alternative is the sharing of virtual pamphlets on the Web and providing links for counseling topics. Human resources however are necessary to evaluate and manage such resources to determine that they are appropriate and up to date.

The National Academic Advising Association Technology in Advising Commission (NACADA) suggests that distance students should have the same advising and counseling resources available to them that the other students have. These include:

- The program provides workshops and/or training in the use of distance education technologies as required for students enrolled in courses/programs.
- The program provides access to the appropriate learning resources as required of distance learning students, i.e., basic skills, course tutorials, disability support, library, etc.
- In order for students to be able to function effectively and achieve academically, they need to be provided with accurate information on the assumptions about the technical competence and skill level required, as well as the actual technical equipment requirements needed to participate.
- The program provides students with accurate and timely information and an internal distance learner network that connects all processes required of the distance learner and provides them with one point of contact for the services listed previously in this chapter.

The NACADA Web site also lists academic advising resources available on the Internet including topics ranging from career counseling to study skills as well as multiple listing of academic advising Web page links to universities across the country. The core values described by the NACADA reflect the fact that advisement is a personal process and establishes a relationship between the students and their institutions. Further, when done correctly, advisement is not just between the student and the advisor but involves a team effort that includes the student support services of the institution, the student, and the advisor. According to the WICHE and NACADA guidelines for developing an advisor's Web page (Carnevale, 2000), the basis for a comprehensive advising site should include the following elements:

1. *A clear and concise explanation of core curriculum (or general education) requirements.* Advisement usually involves a comprehensive explanation of curriculum requirements and a review of what a student has left to complete. Making this information available online will free up some time, will give students greater control and responsibility for the advisement process, and is essential information for students trying to determine course selection if they are unable to meet with an advisor.

2. *A Frequently Asked Questions (FAQ) section.* Every advisor spends a portion of the day repeating answers to the same questions. Putting answers to FAQs online saves time for staff and gives students access to answers as needed.

3. *Informational pages for special populations/self help assistance.* While there are certain common needs among students, there are segments of the population with additional unique concerns. Freshmen, students without declared majors, students on academic probation, and commuters are examples of groups with additional needs for support. Examples of information to include for advisement: career/major information, study skills building worksheets, an explanation of the academic standing policy, information on how to get computer access and technical support, and parking information should on site visits be necessary..

4. *Links to related university sites.* Holistic advisement involves supporting a student both academically and personally. Links to campus services such as student activities calendars, campus organization pages, career services, academic lab locations and hours, and intramural offerings are needed to make sure all needs are being met.

5. *One-on-one access to advisors.* To generate a more personal environment and provide opportunities for interaction, advisors are experimenting with various forms of electronic communications. This is the most critical element in a comprehensive

advising Web site. If advising were simply a matter of giving students a standardized package of information, there would be no reason to have advisors. Access to a qualified advisor can be achieved through the use of chat rooms, listservs, and emails, to mention a few of the most common methods.

The Western Interstate Commission for Higher Education (WICHE) evaluated online student support offerings at 15 colleges and universities and selected what they identified as best practices for integrating technology into student support services. The services evaluated a range from advisement and personal counseling to registration and financial aid. A brief sampling of WICHE's findings include:

- The University of Colorado at Boulder offers the PLUS—personal lookup system. Students can search and register for classes, access grades, apply for financial aid, and explore scholarships (*www.colorado.edu/PLUS/plusguide.html*).
- Washington State University developed a comprehensive online student advising and online advising resource manual. The manual includes 12 main sections covering all aspects of advising from admissions and general education requirements to advising and self-help information (*salc.wsu.edu/Advising/newman/default.asp*).
- Weber State University offers a variety of online student services including e-mail access to an advisor and a career counselor, tutoring, and self-help tips (*wsuonline.weber.edu/advising*).

It should be apparent that student support services cover a broad range of issues that require institutional and faculty resources. If institutions attempt to operate a distance program without addressing these issues, it will soon become apparent that these services are necessary.

FACULTY SUPPORT AND WORKLOAD

Faculty support is another major consideration that institutions need to take into account in support of distance education. The time, knowledge, and skills that are required to design, develop, and teach online cannot be taken for granted or assumed by administrators to be basic faculty skills.

Faculty training for distance education has not traditionally been addressed by university settings. However, as the value and complexity of this endeavor is realized, more institutions are investing time and resources. The Center for Applied Information Technology (CAIT) at Towson University in Towson, Maryland for example, offers faculty training in courseware and multimedia from online instructional designers to technology support staff. Towson has recognized that instructional designers (ID) and instructional technology (IT) support are essential for distance learning success.

The Indiana Higher Education Telecommunication System (IHETS) (2003) recommends that institutions engaged in the delivery of distance learning experiences provide appropriate developmental experiences for their faculty. IHETS suggests that faculty be exposed to various pedagogical strategies that are well-suited to the distance-learning environment, and that exposure to in-services, workshops, and interactions with experienced peers be provided.

Faculty support for course development should also include technical support, to insure that faculty has basic technical skills required to offer online courses. For example, faculty must know how to use e-mail, send attachments, and have a basic understanding of Microsoft Office™ products. More advanced technical skills will be required in the form of using the selected courseware such as Blackboard, Web CT, or Angel. Often university settings that offer online courses also offer training courses for faculty in the use of this software. Other technical support will be required in the form of video or audio recording if lectures are going to be presented using Real Player or similar software.

Faculty workload is a key factor that must be considered and defined. "Faculty workload" is defined as how much a faculty member teaches and how much of his or her work time is taken up with research, administration, and other duties (Hawkins, 1999). The Indiana Higher Education Telecommunication System (IHETS) recommends the development of a system of faculty incentives and rewards to encourage effort and recognize achievement associated with the development and delivery of distance learning courses. IHETS further recommends that there be a mechanism for determining whether distance learning course development and delivery will be included as part of a faculty member's workload or assigned on an overload basis and IHETS further recommends that the institution should define whether special compensation will be provided to faculty members participating in distance learning course development and delivery. The evaluation process according to the IHETS should be in accordance with institutional policy for teaching face-to-face courses.

Intellectual property issues arise around who owns an electronic course once it is created. Does it belong to the institution, faculty member or both? Historically, universities have given copyrights to faculty, allowing them to do as they wish with materials falling under copyright. However, when faculty develop a new invention or process, most campuses defined this creative contribution under their patent policies, because the institution had to commit a significant set of resources, and thus there was a sharing of any benefits derived from this intellectual property (Hawkins, 1999). Similarly, institutions could claim that when a course is developed using universitys software, and university resources, significant institutional resources have been invested thereby creating shared property. Dennis Thompson (1999) claims in his article "Intellectual Property Meets Information Technology", that neither copyright nor patent policy is well suited to dealing with distributed learning materials. He argues that campuses have not defined adequate policies or reached a clear understanding of the issues around intellectual property, conflict of interest, and revenue sharing.

Faculty should also be provided with information regarding copyright laws and course content development for distance learning courses. Just because something is on the Web does not mean that it is there for the taking. The process recommended by IHETS for determining copyright law compliance is as follows:

1. Attention will be paid to the rights and privileges regarding transmission of materials as defined in Section 110(2) of U.S. Copyright Law.
2. If section 110(2) does not apply, "fair use" as defined in Section 107 may apply. The nature and amount of the work

used, and the purpose and effect of the use, will be weighted to determine if fair use applies.

3. If the planned use of a copyrighted work cannot be addressed by Section 110(2) or 107, permission of the content owner may be required.

4. Be aware of how to obtain copyright permission. Some institutions may provide assistance in obtaining such permission.

In addition to providing faculty training for teaching courses online, institutions should also offer faculty training for offering advice to students online. The NACADA suggest standards for faculty as advisors, including:

- A distance education program must provide for appropriate real-time or delayed interaction between faculty, advisors, and students, AND among students.
- The program provides faculty and advisors support to assist students in making informed choices about career and academic goals, self-assessment, decision making, and evaluation of academic career options.
- The program provides faculty and advisors with the support to orient students to the distance-learning environment.
- The institution needs to provide an environment in which faculty as advisors as well as professional advisors can work toward achieving competencies needed to be an advisor of distance learners (Thach & Murphy, 1995).

Although advising is critical for all students, it is even more essential that distance students feel they have a connection to someone at the institution. As these guidelines recommend, if students are to be successful they need more than just quality courses online.

SUMMARY

The importance of institutional commitment from the strategic plan to the home page must be evidenced by faculty support and a sound technological structure. There clearly needs to be a commitment on the part of the institution, the faculty, and the students themselves in order to have a well-supported program of distance courses. When analyzing other institution's guidelines and the various Web resources mentioned throughout this chapter, a checklist could easily be established in order to analyze one's own infrastructure.

REFERENCES

American Distance Education Consortium (ADEC). (2002). Retrieved December 08, 2002, from *http://www.adec.edu/admin/papers/distance-learning_principles.html*.
Association of College and Research Libraries (2002). Retrieved November 24, 2002, from *http://www.ala.org/acrl/guides/distlrng.html*.
Berge, 2 & Schrum, L. (1998). Linking strategic planning with program implementation for distance education. Cause/ Effect 21 (3). Retrieved January 03, 2003 from *http://www.edcause.edu/ir/library/html/cem9836.html*.
Carnevale, D. (2000). Commmissions Web site helps colleges put student services online. The Chronicle of Higher Education. Retrieved January 3, 2003.
Delahoussaye, M., Zemke, R., & Miller, S. (2001). 10 things we know for sure about learning online. *Training,-* 38 (9). (p. 1–8).
Indiana Higher Education Telecommunication System (IHETS) (2003). Retrieved December 16, 2002, from *http://www.ihets.org/learntech/facprinc.html#facwork*.
National Academic Advising Association Technology in Advising Commission (NACADA). Retrieved January 12, 2003, from *http://www.psu.edu/dus/ncta/links.htm*.
Western Cooperative for Telecommunications Education (1999). Retrieved January 3, 2003, from *http://www.wcet.info/resources/publications/guide/guide.htm*.
Hawkins, B. (1999). Distributed learning and institutional restructuring. *Educom Review,* 34(4), 12—17.
Thach E. & Murphy, K. (1995). Competencies for distance education professionals. Educational Technology Research and Development. 43(1). 57–79.
Thompson, D (1999). Intellectual property meets information technology, *Educom Review,* 34(2), 14–21.

APPENDIX A: U.S. COPYRIGHT AND FAIR USE LAW

The following are not infringements of the provisions of Section 106, Copyright Law:

1. Performance or display of a work by instructors or pupils in the course of face-to-face teaching activities of a nonprofit educational institution, in a class-room or similar place devoted to instruction, unless, in the case of a motion picture or other audiovisual work, the performance, or the display of individual images, is given by means of a copy that was not lawfully made under this title, and that the person responsible for the performance knew or had reason to believe was not lawfully made;

2. Performance of a nondramatic literary or musical work or display of a work, by or in the course of a transmission, if- (A) the performance or display is a regular part of the systematic instructional activities of a governmental body or a nonprofit educational institution; and (B) the performance or display is directly related and of material assistance to the teaching content of the transmission; and (C) the transmission is made primarily for (i) reception in classrooms or similar places normally devoted to instruction, or (ii) reception by persons to whom the transmission is directed because their disabilities or other special circumstances prevent their attendance in classrooms or similar places normally devoted to instruction, or (iii) reception by officers or employees of governmental bodies as a part of their official duties or employment.

LIMITATIONS ON EXCLUSIVE RIGHTS OF SECTION 106: FAIR USE

Notwithstanding the provisions of sections 106 and 106A, the fair use of a copyrighted work, including such use by reproduction in copies or phono records or by any other means specified by that section, for purposes such as criticism, comment, news reporting, teaching (including multiple copies for classroom use), scholarship, or research, is not an infringement of copyright. In determining whether the use made of a work in any particular case is a fair use, the factors to be considered shall include:

1. the purpose and character of the use, including whether such use is of a commercial nature or is for nonprofit educational purposes;
2. the nature of the copyrighted work;
3. the amount and substantiality of the portion used in relation to the copyrighted work as a whole; and the effect of the use upon the potential market for or value of the copyrighted work.
4. The fact that a work is unpublished shall not itself bar a finding of fair use if such finding is made upon consideration of all the above factors.

4

Technologies and Competencies Needed for Online Learning

There are numerous technologies that can be and are used for distance education in the health care field. This chapter will investigate four types of technology utilized; the competencies educators and student nurses need to take advantage of those technologies, and resources for further learning.

Distance education implies a separation between the student and the teacher. With the least complex arrangement, distance education in nursing can be demonstrated by a correspondence-type course where written communication is the only interaction between the student and the teacher. At the most complex configuration, it is possible to enroll in a series of courses leading to a degree and never enter the campus nor meet the instructors face to face.

There is a great variety of technology that is used today in the educational setting to educate nurses at the associate, baccalaureate, master's, and doctoral levels. Excelsior College (formerly known as Regents College) in Albany, New York has educated over forty thousand nurses at the associate and baccalaureate levels since its inception in 1971. Students may demonstrate their expertise in various areas by taking proficiency examinations at sites around the United States. The nurses take online courses at home from a variety of schools to fill in gaps in their learning and prepare for the examinations. They may take two-day, interactive workshops around the country to fulfill their requirements. At the graduate level, the nurse may complete the Master of Science in Nursing Administration course almost entirely online.

The only part of the 44–credit degree that is not online is a two-day on-site seminar as part of the capstone course. The first graduates of the online Master of Science in Nursing program at Excelsior graduated in 2002. The Associate, Baccalaureate and Master of Science degree programs in nursing at Excelsior College are accredited by the National League for Nursing Accrediting Commission (NLNAC) that attests to the quality of the programs.

The technologies employed in distance education fall into the major categories of print, data, voice, and video. Prior to selecting a delivery system in which to conduct or take a course, the needs of the learners and the content of the course need to be determined. In some organizations others will dictate the technology and in some cases the instructor is allowed to select the technology. Distance learning can occur in real time (synchronous), a delayed (asynchronous) approach, or a blend of the two. Distance learning can be any combination of the technologies listed below.

PRINT TECHNOLOGY IN DISTANCE EDUCATION

Print media is an inexpensive, low technology approach that can be developed quickly for a distance education course. This technology includes textbooks, journal articles, study guides, workbooks, course syllabi, and case studies.

DATA TECHNOLOGY IN DISTANCE EDUCATION

This category broadly refers to facsimile (fax), real-time computer conferencing, and World Wide Web applications like computer learning systems. It can also encompass the use of electronic mail (e-mail).

VOICE TECHNOLOGY IN DISTANCE EDUCATION

This technology includes telephone, voice mail, audio conferencing, and short-wave radio in addition to audiotapes and the radio.

VIDEO TECHNOLOGY IN DISTANCE EDUCATION

Video technology involves the use of satellites, still images (slides), moving images (film, videotape), and real-time moving images combined with audio conferencing (one-way or two-way video with two-way audio).

THE FOCUS ON COMPUTER MANAGED LEARNING

The World Wide Web is a popular mechanism used in nursing education at a distance. Courses can be self-paced (individuals moving through the course at their own pace) or cohort (a group moving at the same pace).

There are many popular course management systems used in the health care arena today. Among the more popular ones are WebCT, BlackBoard, and Lotus Learning Space. Some schools have the expertise to develop their own online course delivery tools tailored to the individual school. A school can either purchase the software for installation at the school or purchase the use of the software over the www Internet. There are common functionalities within the course management systems. Most courses have similar components:

1. Course communication features—discussion board, chat, e-mail, and a collaborative whiteboard.
2. Course assessment—tests of different kinds can be administered. Other assignments can be distributed, either at the beginning of the course or just before needed. Models of excellent work can be posted as an exemplar to other students.
3. Course management—online grade book, course rosters, student access tracking, and student password information are the usual tools.
4. Course information—syllabus, instructor home page, calendar, course announcements, and task lists. The home page may include facilitator office hours (physical and virtual), course topics to be covered, textbook purchasing information, course objectives, and grading policies. A link to the facilita-

tor e-mail and telephone number should be provided. Links to discussion groups and online forums that students can use to report problems or provide biographical information and a picture should be present. Materials in the classroom can be posted as Web pages or downloadable files (such as Microsoft® PowerPoint™ handouts). Reference material will include bibliographies and articles or perhaps a link to a virtual library.

5. Course didactic features—file uploading and downloading (for example moving MicroSoft® Powerpoint™, MicroSoft® Word™, MicroSoft® Excel™, etc. documents), streaming video and audio, external web links, and course module builders.

COMPARISON OF ONLINE DELIVERY SYSTEMS

A team searching for an appropriate online delivery system can use sources on the Web to compare features of the various products. For example, the Marshall University, WV site offers a comparison at: *http://www.marshall.edu/it/cit/webct/compare/comparison.html.* Sites are available that evaluate a single product.

There are about a dozen online delivery systems available. Some schools have elected to develop their own learning management systems but the majority purchase packaged products. When selecting a system, one might first determine if software is used elsewhere on the campus. Technical support, maintenance, and software fees, etc. can be shared if the same system is purchased. If the School of Nursing is embarking upon the initial effort to find a system, first the assessment of needs must be conducted. Then the software is found which satisfies those needs, followed by the hardware that supports the software.

A chart can be developed to compare the needs of the School of Nursing and the features of the online delivery systems. Some of the school's needs may be to create and grade essay tests or to support faculty in designing the learning space. Each school has different needs and the needs determine what the school will require of the software package. Some requirements (*http://www.marshall.edu*) are listed here:

Instructor Tools

- Online Grading
- Online Testing
- Electronic Mail
- Course Planning
- Course Management
- Student Tracking
- Design Support

Instructional Features

- Synchronous learning space
- Asynchronous learning space
- Faculty able to change content

Student Tools

- Chat Rooms
- Glossary
- Online help

Technical Support

- Security in course

Administrative Tools

- Crash recovery methods

The most well known software packages are:

- Blackboard (*http://www.blackboard.com*)
- WebCT (*http://www.webct.com*)
- Lotus Learning Space (*http://www.lotus.com*)

The features of each software package are described on their Web-sites.

STUDENT REQUIREMENTS

The student needs to have a computer with access to the Internet through an internet service provider in order to access the course. Passwords are used in order to identify the student. There are tutorials available for the various course management systems in order to help the student experience the various course features (i.e., *http://otel.uis.edu/bbtutorial/*). Also there are Web sites that can help the student identify their readiness for taking a course online (*http://www.edu/self_assesment.asp*).

See the University of Maryland School of Nursing site *www.nursing.umaryland.edu/de/frame.htm* or Figure 4.1 for an example of Technical Requirements and Technical Assistance available to the students and facilitators. At the University of Maryland School of Nursing, the entire RN to BSN program as well as the Post Masters Certificate in Nursing Informatics are offered via the Web. Note that the requirements also link users to a Web site where they can download a product and an e-mail to obtain further assistance. The UMNet account refers to school supported electronic mail. Students may take an on-site orientation to online learning or a "virtual" orientation is available on the Web site. In the virtual orientation the student selects an icon for further information on a specific area like "Access and Information about Blackboard." There are also tools to assess whether or not an online course is right for the learner and whether or not technical skills are appropriate. As there is no reliability and validity of the instruments

Please note the following minimum technical requirements for your personal computer (PC):

- Internet Access provided through your Internet Service Provider (ISP) - use at least 56k modem or higher;
- UMnet Account - if you don't have a *UMnet account,* please complete and fax the *request for a UMnet account* form to 410-706-7238
- **E-Mail Account** - an active *UMnet account* is required
- **PC Hardware** - should have at least Pentium 200 or Mac OS 7;
- **Peripherals** - attach a sound card and set of speakers;
- **Browsers** - download and install the latest version of either *Netscape Communicator* or *Internet Explorer 5* (*preferred). Be sure to check your *Java* and *Cache* settings
- **Real Player 8 Basic** - download and *install* the **free** version at *www.real.com*
- **Adobe Acrobat Reader** - download and install at *adobe products*
- **Microsoft Office 2000** - available to currently enrolled UMB students for *only $25*

Figure 4.1 Sample Technical Requirements for University of Maryland School of Nursing Online Courses.

presented, they should be used as general guidelines only. For fun, see *www.marylandonline.org/prospective_students/assess/online_learning_ for_me* which is purported to assess whether or not online learning is appropriate and *www.marylandonline.org/prospective_students/assess/ tech_savvy* to assess the level of technological skills possessed.

Duquesne University School of Nursing, in Pittsburgh, Pennsylvania, offers graduate level courses online including the doctoral degree (*www.nursing.duq.edu/sononline.html*) that started in the online format in 1997. The systems use instructor-mediated technology and a limited on campus requirement.

INFORMATICS COMPETENCIES

The nurse at all levels must have some expertise using information technology at the job site and in an educational setting. Both the course instructor and the student must have basic computer competencies in order to create, maintain, facilitate, and take an online course. Staggers, Gassert, and Curran (2001) studied minimal competencies that nurses must possess. There are 31 competencies identified at the beginning nurse level, as well as fundamental information management and computer technology skills. Examples of these skills are as follows:

- Uses telecommunication devices (i.e., modem, other devices) to communicate with other systems (i.e., access data, upload, download).
- Uses e-mail (e.g., create, send, respond, use attachments).
- Uses presentation graphics (e.g., PowerPoint) to create slides, displays.
- Uses multimedia presentations.
- Uses word processing.
- Demonstrates keyboarding (i.e., typing) skills.
- Uses spreadsheets.
- Uses networks to navigate systems (e.g., files servers, World Wide Web).
- Is able to navigate Windows (e.g., manipulate files using file manager, determine active printer, access installed applications, create and delete directories).

INSTRUCTOR COMPETENCIES FOR ONLINE LEARNING

Teaching in an online learning environment is different from teaching in the traditional classroom. The instructor has to overcome potential barriers caused by technology, time, and place to create an optimal environment for achieving educational goals. The instructor/facilitator must make sure the course is running smoothly and that barriers (that will certainly happen) are overcome quickly. It is important to make the technology as transparent as possible and should be viewed as a tool to enable learning the content of the course.

The instructor must be offered some level of training. For example, if an instructor has utilized Lotus Learning Space® and the school is changing platforms to WebCT®, perhaps only a written handout is needed pointing out the differences in the two software packages. The instructor must know some file management techniques and tips such as transferring files, adding attachments, basic hypertext markup language (HTML), word processing, initiating chats, finding a file in a hierarchical system, and printing files. It is helpful to be able to use spreadsheet and presentation software (like MicroSoft Powerpoint®), and to possess basic skills with database software, as well as know about basic security controls. The more the educator knows about the technical workings of the course management system, the more control he or she has over the course. The educator may elect to learn software tools for developing the home page such as HTML and Dreamweaver, or MicroSoft FrontPage® Protocols such as FTP (file transfer protocol can be used) to upload and download files to and from the students.

One technique utilized to develop a course is the idea of "storyboarding." It is a concept that results in a graphic depiction of a narrative. The course developer starts with an outline of the content for the module and sketches out the module. The graphic could include the screen layout with headings, text, and graphics and navigational controls.

COLLABORATION WITH INFORMATION TECHNOLOGY STAFF

Selecting and using technology is best undertaken as a team effort between students, faculty, support staff, and administration. There are multiple considerations for selecting technology:

1. Hardware considerations (memory, internet connection, lease or purchase a server).

2. Software considerations (MicroSoft PowerPoint®, Real Player)
3. Choosing a teaching platform (WebCT (webct.com), Blackboard (www.blackboard.com), Lotus Learning Space, Outlook Express used by the University of Phoenix, and others)
4. The importance of backup in case of down time
5. Cost and ongoing support considerations.

INSTRUCTIONAL TECHNOLOGY HELP RESOURCES

Technical assistance must be available for both the students and the faculty. Ideally a support facility should be open 24 hours a day, seven days a week. If the support center is not open at all hours, there should be a mechanism to leave both voice and electronic mail messages with a fast response. Typical problems that occur primarily at the start of the course include hardware, software, and network problems. The school of nursing may have designated   support staff in information technology. If the school is part of a larger college or university, support might be obtained from the other departments.

For help with instructional technology there are several Web-based resources such as glossaries of terms posted by the American Society for Training & Development (ASTD) (*http://www.learningcircuits.org/glossary.html*) and Webopedia (*www.webopedia.com*). Specific to nursing is an electronic mailing list hosted by the University of Maryland Baltimore called e-LeaRN. To subscribe, send a note to *listproc@list.umaryland.edu.* In the body of the message type: subscribe e-LeaRN Susan Newbold   (substitute yourfirstname yourlastname). With the welcome message there will be further instructions.

SUMMARY

This chapter has investigated four types of technology that can be utilized in distance education, the competencies educators and student nurses need to take advantage of those technologies, and resources for further learning.

REFERENCES

Blackboard. Retrieved June 15, 2003 from: *http://www.blackboard.com*.

Lotus LearningSpace. Retrieved February 27, 2003 from *http://www.lotus.com/products/learnspace.nsf/wdocs/homepage*.

Staggers, N., Gassert, C. A., & Curran, C. (2001). Informaticscompetencies for nurses at four levels of practice. *Journal of Nursing Education, 40*(7), 303—316.

WebCT. Retrieved June 15, 2003 from *http://www.webct.com*.

5

Reconceptualizing the Online Course

The stage between making the decision to use online learning strategies and actually developing the learning environment is most important and pertinent. Reconceptualizing the learning material means going from "OK, I have this learning material" to using online pedagogy, infrastructure, and technology to make decisions about how the learning material will be presented online. Reconceptualizing is a series of if-then statements. It is a decision tree in which strengths, purpose, and resources are examined to make a decision about the best approach to present the learning material. Reconceptualizing is answering questions and using the answers to guide the development of online learning and communication environments.

The decision tree in Figure 5.1 will guide your decision making. The tree comprises questions, possible answers, and possible actions. These questions were developed using the Guidelines for the Use of Distance Technology in Nursing Education, an appendix of the AACN (1997) White Paper; *Distance Technology in Nursing Education.* Questions will be posed about institutional issues, technology, faculty, and students. Possible answers to the questions are given, and action based on each of the possible answers is proposed.

USING THE DECISION TREE

The following is an example of how answering these questions can guide your decisionmaking. A school of nursing is considering on-

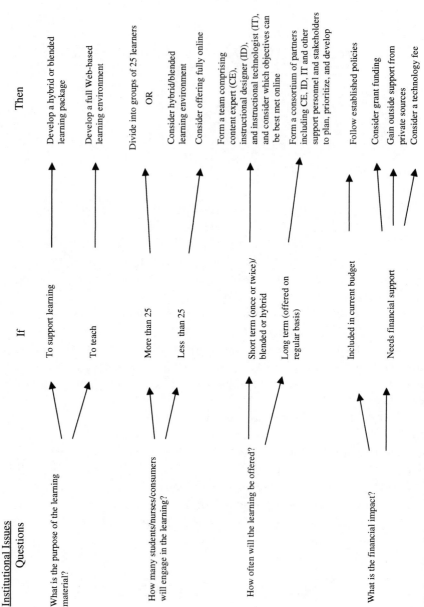

FIGURE 5.1 Decision tree to reconceptualize learning online.

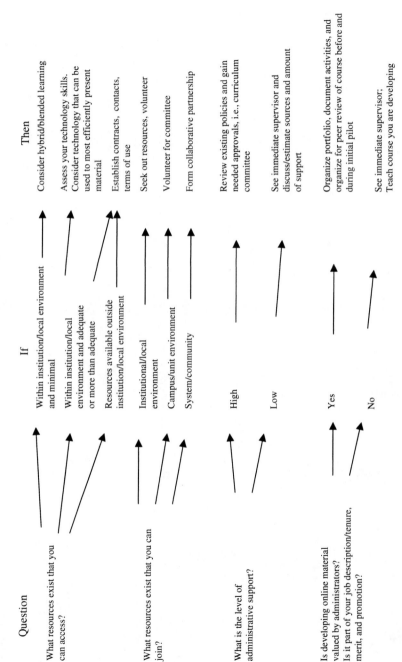

FIGURE 5.1 *(continued)*.

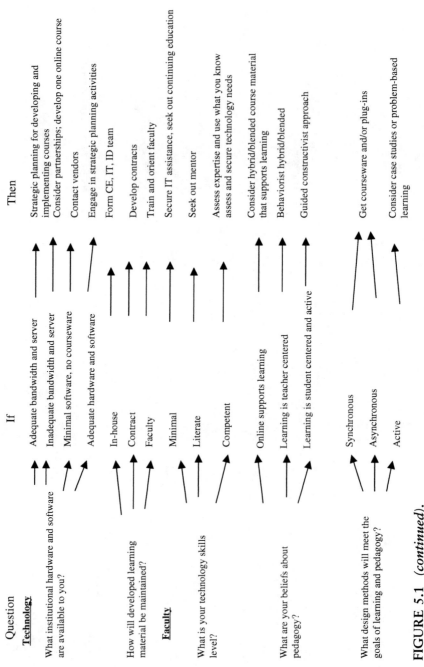

FIGURE 5.1 (*continued*).

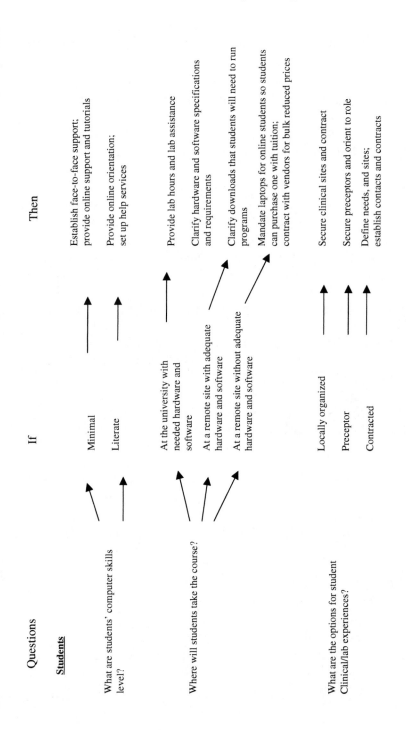

FIGURE 5.1 *(continued)*.

line courses. The dean meets with a department chair and a faculty member, Dr. G., who has experience in teaching online, to discuss the feasibility of moving the RN to BSN program online. The school has a strategic plan that includes online learning. The strategic plan was developed with input from faculty. This information about institutional factors leads to the conclusion that support for online programs is strong. The Dean is willing to provide an information technology (IT) expert and instructional design (ID) support. The program will enroll more than 25 students, and will be long term. The current budget will support development activities. No policies about online courses are available. The school has its own server and enough bandwidth for a limited number of courses. One instructional designer is available for consultation, but no maintenance support personnel are available. The school has three year old desktop computers for faculty members. Microsoft Office, Front Page and Dreamweaver are available. Several laptops are available to faculty and all computers have Internet access. Computer laboratories are available for students with over 50 terminals in the school of nursing. Dr. G. has been involved in a project to guide and mentor faculty to teach online for a year. She is computer literate and is a content expert (CE) in community health nursing. She believes that students learn throughinteracting with learning material and that students can learn from each other. Dr. G. believes that the faculty motivates and guides learning. She would like to provide a variety of learning options for students. Dr. G. would like to include course content, bulletin boards for discussions, small groups for students to complete activities, and synchronous chat rooms for office hours. She would like student assessment to include participation in discussions, assignments, and exam grades. Students should have computers available for use outside the school of nursing.

DECISIONS

Based on this information, one course in the RN to BSN program would be developed at the beginning. This course would have a community focus and Dr. G. will develop and teach it. Teaching the course would be included in her workload and developing the course would be considered "service" and included as a "merit" activity. The current instructional designer would contract with a courseware vendor and would teach Dr. G. how to use the courseware. Dr. G. would partner with a technical person (IT) and the two would work as a CE and IT team. The course would be organized by modules. Each module would have objectives, readings, content, small-group activities, and large-group discussion questions. Content would be disseminated in written and voice formats. Grading would include projects, participation, and exams.

The course was marketed prior to and at course registration and students registered in the usual way. The names of the registered students were sent to Dr. G and she entered the students into her online course. While the pilot was in process, the faculty administrator for the undergraduate program, Dr. G., and the Instructional Designer met to plan for future courses. Evaluation information from the pilot course was solicited several times during the course and at the end of the course and was used to refine the course and to design other courses. One new course per faculty member was added each semester for a year. The lessons learned were shared with faculty who were developing their courses. The team guided and supported new faculty developing courses and teaching online. Faculty new to teaching online were invited to join the Web-based Teaching Committee and the team grew each semester. Sharing ideas and experiences with peers was essential for the development of the program. Through this group, policies, online student registration and support, student and faculty support systems were developed.

Another scenario might be is high support and minimal faculty skill. If the faculty is motivated and willing to learn to develop online courses, go online. If there is moderate support and high resources, go online. If there is minimal support and resources, consider hybrid or blended courses and build support and stakeholders. A hybrid or blended course combines technology and traditional classroom strategies.

Developing is an excellent way to begin while gathering resources, support, and experience. Gravitate toward a level at which the effort will be successful. Maximize the resourcesavailable and incorporate new resources and technology that will enhance your course. Pilot the material, have the material peer reviewed, and solicit learner feedback frequently for incorporation into course revisions.

RECONCEPTUALIZING COURSES

Hybrid or Blended Courses

The decision to put a portion of the course material online is made. This is called blended learning. Driscoll (2002) defines blended learning as augmenting traditional face-to-face learning with technology. It is also defined as the mixing of technology with job tasks to create a seamless transition between learning and working.

> Blended learning is a great way to initiate an organization into e-learning because it benefits learners, the training staff, and the organization's bottom line. It allows organizations to gradually move learners from traditional classrooms to e-learning in small steps, making change easier to accept. Working in a blended environment enables instructors and instructional designers to develop the skills needed for e-learning in small increments. Training professionals can move small sections online as the needed e-learning skills are developed. Many organizations have spent a great deal of money developing classroom materials and are not about to throw that investment away. Blended learning allows organizations to supplement or complement existing courseware rather than replace it (Driscoll, 2002, p. 1).

What might be some options for blended learning? Look at the learning goals and objectives, the available technology, and the skill level of the faculty. Think about maximizing the use of technology to create the most effective environment for student learning. Some of the options are described below:

- Use voice, video, and/or text to put the essential content online and use class time for discussion activities and case studies. For example, use MicroSoft PowerPoint and Real-

Player and narrate some psychiatric or didactic nursing class-es to create a mini-lecture. Limit content to a specific unit of study, for example, depression. Give essential knowledge on depression that will accomplish the objectives. The learning material should be limited to about twenty minutes (consid-ering "buffering" which may lengthen the time to complete viewing the material and student ability to attend to the content. Buffering is the transfer of large multi-media files from a server to a local computer in a viewable format). The required reading on depression and the minilecture on depression should be completed before class. Use in-class time for small group discussion of case studies. The case studies will help the student to begin to apply the content. Use the scenario of depression in a teenager, a post-partum woman, and/or an adult. Careplans can be the outcome of the case study.

- Use class time to impart content and use online environ-ments to support learning through links relevant to the learn-ing material.
- Use online support for administrative and organizational functions such as grading, computerized examinations, an-nouncements, directions, and syllabus presentation.
- Use the online environment for discussion of case studies. Set up a discussion forum for each case study or divide the students into small groups to discuss the case study and develop careplans.

MENTAL MODELS

The decision to present the learning material totally online is made. The next step is to develop plans that will maximize what is known, the resources available, and the "lowest common denomi-nator" of student hardware and software. It is more effective to use what is available to its optimal capacity and use what is known to the fullest potential to produce a learning environment that will maximize assets. The "lowest common denominator" means that not all students have access to the same hardware and software or bandwidth. If a course is built using software that the student does not have or does not have access to, the student will become frustrated and dissatisfied. For example, when using a minilecture requiring plug-ins for viewing multimedia or audio files, the content of this minilecture may not be available to students with older computers or slow dial-up connections. Providing content using links and text will provide information to a larger audience because it is a lowest common denominator and the most accessible to students.

How can the course instructor convert traditional learning material to an online learning environment? What may be used to create the online learning environment? These are the next questions in reconceputaling learning environments for a Web-based format. Traditional classroom teaching differs from online teaching it they uses different learning modalities.

Because of the lack of visual feedback from students (shaking of heads while you are lecturing or closed eyes and bobbing heads), online learning environments need to give students a clear picture of what they are learning and how they will learn it. In the traditional classroom the teacher begins a learning session by telling the students what they will learn (learning objectives), gives them the information needed to learn the intended learning (content), and then the teacher summarizes what the students have learned. A traditional teacher begins by saying "Today we are going to learn about depression" and at the end might say, "Let me summarize what we have said about depression," so the student knows where they are in the learning process. In online learning environments, students still need to know where they are in the learning process and this is done through mental models. Mental models give meaning to concepts and promote the transfer of knowledge from the "didactic" to the "real" world.

Example of Reconceptualizing to Online Learning Environments

Let's follow Dr. G. in the reconceptualization process. Dr. G. reconceptualized an undergraduate Community/Public Health Nursing course. She considered her pedagological beliefs that students learn differently and have unique learning styles. She decided to include learning strategies such as text, verbal and discussion modes of learning to accommodate a variety of learning styles. Dr. G. decided to organize by modules. The traditional classroom course was organized by "week"—Week 1, Week 2, etc. The online course includes objectives and readings, content, and small group activities. The content outline looks like this:

Community/Public Health Nursing

Module 1: History of Public/Community Health Nursing
- Objectives and Readings
- Content
- Activities

Module 2: Influences on the Practice of Community/Public Health Nursing
- Objectives and Readings
- Content
- Activities

Module 3: Cultural Influences on the Practice of Community/Public Health Nursing
- Objectives and Readings
- Content
- Activities

Module 4: Care Management
- Objectives and Readings
- Content
- Activities

Module 5: Home Visiting
- Objectives and Readings
- Content
- Activities

Module 6: Program Planning
- Objectives and Readings
- Content
- Activities

Module 7: Environmental Health
- Objectives and Readings
- Content

- Activities

Module 8: Multiproblem Families
- Objectives and Readings
- Content
- Activities

Module 9: Vulnerable Populations
- Objectives and Readings
- Content
- Activities

Module 10: Epidemiology
- Objectives and Readings
- Content
- Activities

Module 11: Organization and Finance of the Public Health Care System
- Objectives and Readings
- Content
- Activities

Module 12: Ethical, Legal, Political, and Research Aspects of Community/Public Health Nursing
- Objectives and Readings
- Content
- Activities

This design was cumbersome and needed streamlining. Dr. G. looked at the content and decided that the course really contained four areas of content: History and Scope, Practice, Focus, and Tools. Dr. G. shifted the modules into four content areas as illustrated in Figure 5.2.

Each section contains several of the original modules. History and Scope comprises modules 1, 2, and 3; Practice comprises modules 4, 5, 6, and 7; Focus comprises modules 8 and 9; Tools comprises modules 10, 11, and 12. The content areas and the modules within that area are presented in the same color and each content area has a different color. Each module contains objectives and readings, minilecture and activities. There are several advantages to this reconceptualization. Students repeatedly see the four content areas and these become the four concepts of Community/Public

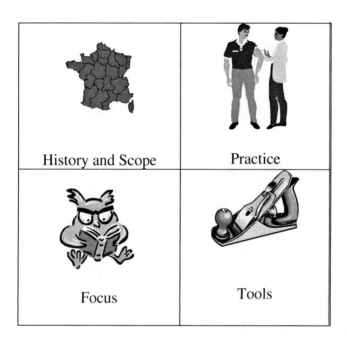

FIGURE 5.2 The reconceptualized community public health nursing course.

Health Nursing. The concepts, called "mental models" are consistently reinforced when the student accesses the course content. Mental models give meaning to concepts and promote the transfer of knowledge from the "didactic" to the "real" world. When the student sees the word "tools" over and over, the student forms a mental model that community/public health nursing has tools and one of those tools is epidemiology (a module).

Operationalizing the mental model in an activity strengthens the impact of the mental model. For example, one of the activities in the "tools" mental model could include a case study of an epidemic of influenza in a community.

Reconceptualizing a course provides the student with a "map" of the course so the student can see what the course is about, where they have been, and where they are going in the course.

PEDAGOGY

First consider pedagological beliefs and think about what can use be used to operationalize those beliefs. Ask yourself the following questions:

- Do you prefer one learning style or many?
- Do you believe that group communication will support learning?
- Do you support synchronous communication?
- Do you support asynchronous communication?

Which technology will be used to create the course is the next question. Some options are voice through RealPlayer, video, links, and text and/or PowerPoint presentations. Start with what is familiar and consider the philosophy of teaching and learning espoused by the instructor.

Example of Reconceptualizing Pedagogy

Consider how Dr. G. operationalizes her philosophical and pedagogical beliefs about teaching and learning online. Dr. G. chose to include minilectures with PowerPoint and voice and voice attached to each slide. The minilecture included content that was pertinent to meeting module objectives and to complete the module activities. The voice scripts were included in printand both the PowerPoint slides and the scripts would be available to students; thus allowing for a wider variety of learning styles using voice and text. Students are divided into small groups to complete module activities. Students post ideas to a discussion board, which contains a question relating each module to the "real" world. An example of a small group activity is as follows: Students are given census data about a geographic community. They also view a video tour of the same community. Students are asked to develop a consensus "composite picture" of the community using both types of data. Dr. G. provides synchronous office hours for one hour a week.

Another consideration is grading. Will participation be graded? If so, how does the student need to participate to earn a grade?

Traditionally, Schools of Nursing are bound by approval of the curriculum committee. Do traditional and online classes have the same syllabus? Must grading be the same with both modalities? If so, how will participation be included in the online learning environment? Is grading of participation necessary to engage students in active communication during the course? Participation can be a mandatory and expected behavior in online courses. Examples of criteria for expected participation and grading can be found in Chapter 7, Course Management Methods, of this book.

Reconceptualizing Laboratory Courses

Since many nursing courses have associated laboratory experiences, consideration must be made for learning psychomotor skills. The component of the learning process for psycho-motor skills that differs in traditional vs. online learning environments is practice and feedback. Traditional learners learn the procedure then attend laboratory sessions to perform the skill under the supervision of an expert who will give the students feedback on their performance. Once they master the skill in the laboratory, the student will perform the skill with a proctor and their proficiency will be evaluated. Another name for this clinical activity is called a "cognitive apprenticeship", which is discussed in further detail in the chapter on interaction. Students learning in online environments can obtain the didactic material online. How can students be provided with practice opportunities and feedback and how can their proficiency be evaluated? Some options are:

- Students attend the laboratory sessions with traditional students.
- Students are assigned preceptors in the community by the course instructor and the preceptor gives feedback to the student.
- Preceptors can be chosen by the student and the instructor coordinates and monitors the experience while the preceptor gives feedback.
- Clinical instructors can be assigned to a geographic cohort of students; the laboratory experience is contracted with

local institutions and the instructor gives feedback to the students.

- Partnerships with Schools of Nursing and contract for their laboratory facilities and instructors to give feedback.
- Contracts with schools near the student that have interactive video options and laboratory facilities; students can practice using procedure guidelines then two-way video to the faculty who can give feedback via television.
- Use laptops with videoconferencing to practice skills with the instructor at a remote location who gives feedback.

Some options for assessing students are:

- Students can take a proficiency test at the school of nursing that is administrated by the instructor.
- The proficiency test can be given and assessed by their preceptor.
- The proficiency test can be administered by a preceptor, videotaped and then assessed by the instructor.
- The student can take the proficiency test at an outreach site where an instructor will administrate and assess students in a geographic cohort.
- Community resources can administer the proficiency test at an outreach site and the instructor assesses student proficiency via live video.
- Students can use a laptop computer and videoconferencing to perform the proficiency test with the instructor assessing from a remote site.

Reconceptualizing Clinical Courses

Some courses that are offered online have a clinical component. Clinical experiences should provide the students with guidance, mentoring, role modeling, feedback, and assessment of clinical competencies associated with the course. The following questions should be asked:

- How will guidance and mentoring be given to the student and by whom?

- Who will provide role modeling and how?
- How will the student receive feedback?
- How will the mastery of course competencies be assessed for each student?

Baier and Mueggenburg (2001) used online learning environments to support clinical instruction by posting travel directions, agency information, and pictures of clinical sites. They included links to clinical agencies and other sites that would be useful to the clinical experience. They asked students to write and e-mail their instructor reflective papers after each clinical day. Students worked together online on group clinical projects. Zimmerman, Barnasun, and Pozehl (1999) encouraged graduate acute care nursing students to take clinicals in their home community. Students were encouraged to have a laptop computer and to take and use their laptop computer in clinical settings. Students used desktop video conferencing to obtain feedback from their instructor who was at a distant location site. Instructors answered questions, observed student performance, and gave feedback while observing student-patientinteractions. Blakeley and Curran-Smith (1998) organized distance education community health nursing clinicals on the east coast of Canada:

> In Newfoundland and Labrador, community health nursing falls under the jurisdiction of six regional community health boards. Support for the new clinical course was, therefore, sought from each region's nursing director. Guidelines were developed outlining the expectations of the community health nurses (CHNs) in relation to distance students. As faculty could not directly supervise the students, CHNs would act as field guides regardless of whether placements were in St. John's or rural communities. The CHNs assigned to the students were called community health nursing "guides" or CHNGs. Each guide received a copy of the guidelines (1998, p. 149–150).

Teleconferences were held every two weeks for 45 minutes each to discuss experiences, assignments, and specific case studies. Each student had access to a teleconferencing site. After the course was over, students, guides, and faculty were asked for feedback. Students responded that the clinical placement was appropriate and provided them with opportunities to learn and integrate new knowledge and skills. The CHNGs asked for more information about the course and their roles and responsibilities. They were willing to provide information about the student but did not want to assign a grade to the student.

Faculty commented on increased workloads. The overall experience was described as worthwhile and challenging.

Some suggestions for providing clinical students with guidance, mentoring, and role modeling are:

- Students enroll in the same clinicals as the traditional students. If students are location bound, other clinical options must be developed.
- Students have a faculty appointed or student found preceptor who acts as a role model and who provides the student with experiences to accomplish the clinical objectives.
- Clustered experiences—instructor arranges for geographically clustered, intensive, i.e., 4–day, 32 to 40 hour experiences for a cohort of students in a specific geographic location.

Video conferencing with the instructor provides student-to-student and student-to-instructor interactions. Logs written by students in location-bound settings and shared with the preceptor and instructor provide information for the instructor to assess student perception and progress toward meeting clinical objectives.

SUMMARY

Reconceptualize the learning environment begins with the decision to transfer traditional course material into anonline learning environment. The process of answering questions about a course and using the answers to guide the development of the online learning and communication environments will helps capitalize on the benefits of the Web and computer technology. Many opportunities exist to enhance an online course through the appropriate application of technology such as multimedia, links, and synchronous and asynchronous discussions. Laboratory and clinical courses are challenges for designing nursing courses in an online format but as the technology advances, current methods of offering these courses can only be improved.

REFERENCES

American Association of Colleges of Nursing (1997). White Paper: Distance Technology in Nursing Education. Retrieved   December 8, 2002, from *www.aacn.nche.edu/Publications/positions/whitepaper.htm*.

Baier, M. & Mueggenburg, K. (2001). Using the internet for clinical instruction. *Nurse Educator, 26*(1).

Blakeley, J.A., & Curran-Smith, J. (1998). Teaching community health nursing by distance methods: Development, process, and evaluation. *The Journal of Continuing Education in Nursing, 29*(4), pp. 148–53.

Driscoll. M. (2002). Blended learning: Let's get beyond the hype. *E-Learning Magazine, www.elearningmag.com/elearning/article/articleDetail. jsp?id=11755*.

Zimmerman, L.M., Barnason, S., & Pozehl, B. (1999). Distance education programs for advanced practice nurses: Questions to ask. *AACN Clinical Issues, 10*(4), pp. 508–514.

6
Designing the Online Learning Environment

Instructional design refers to a systematic and reflective process that translates the principles of learning and instruction into plans for instructional materials, activities, information resources, and evaluation (Smith & Ragan, 1999). Instructional design answers the questions: Where are we going; How will we get there? How will we know when we get there? Smith and Ragan (1999) identified three components in the instructional design process a:

- instructional analysis (Where are we going?)
- instructional strategy (How will we get there?)
- evaluation (How will we know when we get there?)

Instructional analysis includes assessing the learner and developing learning goals and objectives. Instructional strategy includes developing, delivering, and maintaining the methods and strategies for learning. Evaluation includes using strategies to assess the student's progress toward attaining the objectives (Smith & Ragan, 1999). The design should be specific enough that it is easy to implement, but flexible enough to allow faculty to be creative.

Instructional design is based on instructional-design theory, which provides guidance in developing learning environments. "Instructional design theories are design oriented, they describe methods of instruction and the situations in which those methods should be used, the methods can be broken into simpler component methods, and the methods are probabilistic" (Reigeluth, 1999, p. 7). Instructional design is the preparation and production of learning material and includes developing objectives and goals, and formulating teaching and assessment strategies. Educational theory guides design structure.

GUIDED CONSTRUCTIVISM

Guided constructivism is a combination of elements from behaviorist and constructivist theories. Behaviorism is reflected in the use of objectives that are behaviorally stated, measurable, and timed. How does using constructivist theory impact design? Winn (1991) describes three differences between traditional teaching and constructivism: analysis, determinism, and replication. In traditional learning, students learn the parts then synthesize the parts to master the whole (analysis). Constructivists view learning as pieces that are related to other pieces. In traditional learning instructors look at methods of instruction and select a method that is appropriate and congruous with meeting the instructional goals. It is assumed that learning will take place if the appropriate method is used. The appropriate method used to present the learning material is determined by the theory the instructor uses. This implies that theory will predict and that learning is predictable (determinism). Winn (1991) suggests that the people "do not think logically" because they "make decisions on the basis of incomplete information, intuition, experience, hunches, and guesses" (Winn, 1991, p. 199). The constructivist view is that when students are constructing knowledge, learning cannot be predicted. If learning is predictable, then it is replicable. This assumes that methods have similar effects on students and that if a method worked well once, it will work well again. "The assumption that well-designed instruction is replicable is little more than a variant of the assumption that human behavior is predictable" (Winn, 1991, p. 92). The constructivist view is that the construction of knowledge has a different impact on students. Learning (especially complex learning) needs to be delivered in such a way that it can be revisited over and over so it can be viewed in context with other learning. Learning should be dynamic and not predictable.

CONSTRUCTIVIST DESIGN

Winn (1991) suggests designing the learning shell and allowing learning to be flexible so students can move around and notice relationships. Allow students to retrace their steps and to network for the sharing of constructed ideas with others. Learning environments should use an interface that is comfortable for the student and has a legible screen design. The interface should be as transparent as possible.

Honebein (1996) suggests several ideas for designing constructivist learning environments:

1. Provide multiple ideas and experiences so students can compare a variety of solutions and alternative approaches.
2. Represent realistic, authentic, and relevant real-world examples into the online learning environment.
3. Design experiences so the learner can construct knowledge and the instructor can facilitate the knowledge construction.
4. Include reflective activities so the learner can learn and then relearn.
5. Use social interaction to enhance learning.
6. Develop learner-centered experiences so the students feel ownership of the learning process.

In this chapter, guided constructivist theory will be used to design learning environments for nursing. The target population, the purpose, three site delivery designs, navigation, page layout, and interaction will be discussed.

No single design is "right" or "perfect." Boshier Mohapi, Malton, Qayyum, Sadownik, and Wilson (1997) describe criteria of a 'best-dressed' course as one that is accessible and that includes an ease of connection, a positive first impression and a mode of learning. The Web architecture should contain graphics, animation, discussions, chat, student work areas, and links. A 'best-dressed' course has a high face validity in which the instructor posts a photograph and the course has integrity and soundness. The course should be attractive, meaning that there are alluring links, a level of enjoyment, imagination, and friendliness.

Constructivists view learning as student-centered and advocate that learning objectives be developed by the learner. Although this is feasible for many disciplines, it is not always feasible for nursing. Nursing relies on learning objectives that are generated by the instructor. Objectives must be included in the design of nursing courses and will most likely be instructor generated, a characteristic of behaviorist theory.

Combining instructor-driven objectives with the constructivist view results in what is called a guided constructivist view. The design considerations based on the review of the literature will include:

- The target population
- The purpose and objectives
- Site delivery
  - Content
  - Designs
  - Activities
  - Developing multimedia
- Navigation
- Page layout
- Interaction
  - Synchronous
  - Asynchronous
  - Discussion questions

THE TARGET POPULATION

The first step in course design is assessing the learner (the target population), their existing knowledge of the course material, their experience in learning in online environments, and their level of computer competence. For example, a course introducing new students in an undergraduate nursing program to the concepts of health would be structured differently than a senior level course in community health nursing with a clinical component. The new students may be RNs returning to school for the first time in many years and this may be the first online course some learners have taken so they have no experience with learning online. Their technical literacy levels may be low, and they probably do not know other students in the course or program. On the other hand, the senior level students may already have had a required technology course. They may have either taken or heard about online courses from other students so they have a support group, and they may be assigned to a clinical group with a clinical instructor who can answer questions and clarify the content that is learned online. The design for the new student would be more structured with explicit due dates for activities. To increase socialization among new students, small groups might be included so students can share their ideas with five or six other students instead of the larger class. Because participation is so important to the learning process, including a grade for participation in the new student class is a consideration. The discussion questions would be structured differently in each class. The new students may or may not be nurses, so discussion questions might incorporate life experiences that all students can relate to. The new students may be asked to devise a composite picture of a healthy community based on their readings and personal experience, whereas the seniors might be asked to develop a nursing care plan for a multiproblem family or pregnant teens in a community. The RN to BSN students tend to use nursing lingo that the traditional BSN (non-RN) student may not understand. In a virtual chat discussion about using the Health Belief Model to develop a colon cancer prevention program, the RNs may be discussing colonoscopies and the non-RNs are asking, "What's that?" If the new student class comprises all RN to BSN students, the activities can be devised to incorporate nursing experience. Ask yourself who the learners are, what their experiences with online learning are, and what they know about the learning material.

Assessing learning style is also important for the designer and the learner. The instructor or course designer can provide a variety of learning activities that address the different modes of learning. The Illinois Online Network (ION, n.d.) offers a learning style quiz that can be taken to assess the primary learning style. Learners can take the test to determine their style. Included in the course should be directions for students to use specific learning activities based on their style. The Illinois Online Network (ION, n.d.) describes several learning styles and learning preferences. The visual/verbal learner may prefer to read learning material. The visual/nonverbal learner may prefer to learn from graphs and diagrams. The auditory/verbal learner may prefer to hear the learning material. The tactile/kinesthetic learner may prefer to learn through hands-on experiences (ION, n.d.).

Consideration should be given to how the learner moves through the learning experience. Learning can be self-paced where the learner independently progresses through the learning experiences. Learners can be admitted to a series of courses or learning experiences at the same time (as a cohort). The cohort takes courses on the same schedule and ends the courses at the same time. Consider which will be most effective for your learners.

THE PURPOSE

The objectives should be stated in measurable terms and should be succinct in communicating what the student will accomplish by the end of the learning experience. Objectives should be learner and content appropriate. Objectives for the course may be outlined in the course syllabus. These broad objectives should be broken down into manageable objectives for the learning content. For example, a course objective may be that the learner will plan, implement, and evaluate a smoking cessation program in a community group. In the module, the objective is broken down into smaller objectives, for example "the learner will describe the process of developing an implementation plan" or "the learner will define formative evaluation."

In 1995 the Innovations in Distance Education (Innovations) project funded by the AT&T Foundation was launched at Pennsylvania State University. In this project, faculty worked in teams to examine issues related to the design and development of distance education programs. The outcome was "An Emerging Set of Guiding Principles and Practices for the Design and Development of Distance Education." The guiding principles for learning goals and content presentation are:

1. Learning goals are part of the instructional design plan.
2. Specific instructional strategies and activities should be directed toward providing learners with the necessary skills, knowledge and experience to meet the goals and objectives of the course.
3. Assessment of performance should be directed toward measuring the learning goals.
4. Faculty should be provided with the instructional design and development support they need to create and prepare instructional materials for delivery via distance education.

SITE DELIVERY

The site delivery structure is dependent on the content and the learners, and answers the question: What is the best way to present the content for our learners to learn? There is no right or wrong method but what is important is having a rationale for making decisions.

Content

Content is the information the learner needs to know to successfully achieve the objectives. Considering that learners have many differing learning styles, the content should be presented using many different strategies. You may question, "Why?" The answer is, that "we can!" We can easily present content using different formats. Some examples of instructional formats to present content are: audio tapes, newspaper or journal articles, movie clips, video, guest speakers, interactive software, links, interview, or text-based materials.

Content should be broken down into "chunks" and organized. The basic steps in organizing your information are to divide it into logical units, establish a hierarchy of importance and generality, use the hierarchy to structure relationships among chunks, then analyze the functional and aesthetic success of your system (Webstyle guide, 2002). Chunks should be logical and should organize the content. Two examples of chunks are modules and units.

The chunks of information are organized into a flexible and logical format, and then they are organized into mental models.

Mental models show the learner what they are learning, where they are in the course, and the relationship of each chunk in the course to other chunks. For example, an undergraduate course in gerontological nursing maybe divided into chunks called modules, for example:

Module 1   Introduction to the aging process
Module 2   Theories of aging
Module 3   Physical, psychological, sociological, and spiritual aspects of aging
Module 4   Common health problems
Module 5   Assessing the client
Module 6   Assessing the family
Module 7   Interventions: needs and resources
Module 8   Legal issues related to aging
Module 9   Ethical issues related to aging

These chunks should be organized into mental models. One idea is to combine modules 1 to 3 into a section that could be called "The aging process" Modules 4 to 7 could be called "Caring for the aging client and family". Another section could be "Considerations in nursing care" (modules 8 and 9). The mental models could be the aging process, caring for aging clients and considerations in nursing care. When the learner is navigating to module 1, the learner must pass through "the aging process," thus illustrating where the learner is in the course and what is next in the course. The repetition of the mental models will instill in the student that in gerontology nursing, the nurse assesses and implements nursing care with the client and family and there are characteristics of the aging process and legal and ethical issues that should be considered in nursing care. The graphic is illustrated in Figure 6.1.

Designs

Once the content is conceptualized, the next step is to decide how to structure the course. Three site structures are: The Spread, The Checklist, and The Linear Mode with Star Nodes Attached.

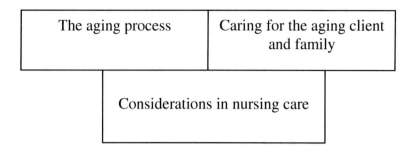

FIGURE 6.1 The reconceptualized course.

THE SPREAD

ALN (2000) describes *The Spread* (Figure 6.2) as a typical design. Course material is linked from the home page so it is easy to navigate, but this design can be cluttered if there is a large amount of content.

The advantage of *The Spread* is that it is organized to present discrete chunks of information and it provides a predetermined structure that will guide the learner through the learning environment. This design supports sequential learning and "it allows global learning with access to all of the instructional materials. It also adds a structure that will help novice users navigate the materials"

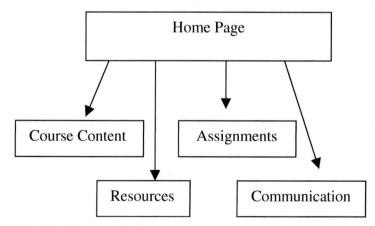

FIGURE 6.2 The spread.

(Learning to Learn, n.d.). A disadvantage is that navigating is limited to forward and backward with the home page as the organizing point.

THE CHECKLIST

ALN (2000) calls *The Checklist* design an orderly sequence of learning material. It is a simple, linear model that works well with basic content.

Unit 1   (Unit 1 — Unit 2 — Unit 3 — Unit 4)
Unit 2
Unit 3
Unit 4

The advantage of this design is that it is orderly and presents material in a learning sequence. The disadvantage is that navigating to the end of the sequence is time consuming. Additionally, this linear format does not support the student who chooses to move around within the content since Unit 2 is usually based on information in Unit 1, and so on.

THE LINEAR MODE WITH STAR NODES ATTACHED

The Linear Mode With Star Nodes Attached (Figure 6.3) allows for an organized, sequential flow of information while providing an unstructured, webbed format so that the learner can access sites in any order through a central point, the home page. The advantage of the *Linear Mode With Star Nodes Attached* is that it allows for both structured and global learning. The disadvantage is that content should be posted weekly to keep the student focused (Learning to Learn, n.d.).

Activities

Activities support learner progression through the content material. Activities should include real world experiences and active learning strategies. Some activities are: case studies, group or individual

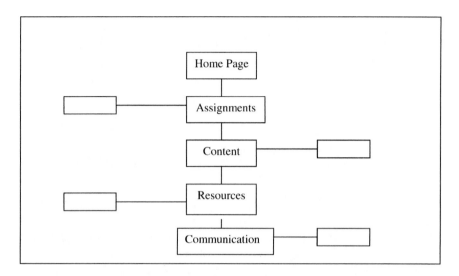

FIGURE 6.3 The Linear Mode with Star Nodes Attached design model.

projects, peer interaction through discussion, and active learning strategies such as collaborative problem solving or Web quests.

Multimedia

The use of multimedia presentations is resource and experience driven. Most instructors stay with what they know and what they have because, in general, instructors do not have the time or technical skill to develop their own multimedia presentations. Little or no information is in the literature to give guidance as to whether a multimedia presentation is more effective than a text-based presentation of content. However, it does offer an alternative way of learning for those students who prefer audio presentations.

The guiding principles suggested by IDE (Innovations, n.d.) for instructional media and tools are:

1. Instructional media and tools should support the predetermined learning goals and objectives of the learning program.
2. The technology that is used should be appropriate for the widest range of students within that program's target audience.

3. Technology should clearly enhance learning.
4. The technology used should be adequately prepared and supported in order to maximize the capabilities of instructional media and tools.
5. The design used should reflect the diversity of potential learners.
6. A systematic design model should be used to guide the selection and application of media and tools.
7. Contingency strategies for technology-related interruptions must be in place.

The general rule of thumb is that "less is more". In other words, instructors can sometimes overuse technological enhancements, which end up not enhancing the course or content at all. If overused or used incorrectly, multimedia presentation can be distracting. Animation, for example, can be effectively used to demonstrate the flow of blood through the chambers of the heart, but it can also be used inappropriately causing your course to resemble a Las Vegas billboard.

NAVIGATION

Using the three-click rule will help with organizing the flow of information. Get the learner where you want them to go in three clicks of the mouse. Navigation directions can be in the form of graphic, picture, or text (See examples in Figure 6.4). Regardless of whether one, or the other, or both are used, be consistent and place the same thing in the same location on every page. Whether it is text along the left side of the page, or text boxes strung across the bottom of the page, or icons in the center of the page and text at the bottom, continue this pattern on every page. The home link is most important in

    HOME

FIGURE 6.4 Navigational graphic or picture, navigational text.

navigation because it gets the learner back to a central place. Brueckner (1999) offers the following "do not's":

- **Do NOT overuse bolding. It causes confusion.**
- Do not use the color blue to emphasize text because blue is associated with hypertext.
- Do not use more than 3 different fonts, because it may **confuse the learner**.

PAGE LAYOUT

The layout of each page should be consistent, appropriate in look and
feel, and have a user-friendly interface (Learning to Learn, n.d.). Consistency means using the same layout on each page and that includes
color, background, fonts, headings, text layout and navigation cues.
The graphic design should be fun, professional, simple, high-tech, and
slick. The design is a reflection of the organization and should be
professional, but it should also be functional and easy to use. Too
much information on a page can make the page look cluttered and can
interfere with what the learner should learn. Ask yourself how each
piece of information on a page will help the learner learn.

The basic page layout includes links that are color coded and positioned in the same place on every page. Each page should have a title
at the top that describes what is on the page. The bottom of the page
should have a link to the person responsible for the Web page, explain-
ing when it was created and where it is located (Brueckner, 1999).
Brueckner offers these additional tips:

- Use headings, bolding, bullets, and graphics to emphasize im-
portant information.
- Use consistent groupings, ordering, and labeling.
- Group information into logical units.
- Look at each page in the same way the learner will see it so
you can visualize the flow of information.

The home page should include information that the learner needs to
begin the learning process. The vital information that should be on the

home page is: a link to course information; instructor name, contact information and a picture; a welcome message from the instructor either in text or streaming audio; and the required textbook and how to obtain it (ALN, 2000).

INTERACTING

Synchronous interaction requires participation with others at the same time, for example chat rooms and audio or video conferencing. Asynchronous interactions are not time-dependent, for example, bulletin boards or electronic mail lists.

Students should have four types of asynchronous interactions (Learning to Learn, n.d.). There should be a forum in which learners can introduce themselves. The forum can be based on a general question such as "What would you like to tell us about yourself," or more specific, such as "When did you realize that you wanted to be a nurse?" for first-year nursing students. The introductory forum provides an opportunity for learners to find out what they have in common. If it is possible, learners should provide a picture of themselves. The instructor should always provide a picture. These activities enhance bonding and start building learning communities. The second forum is to obtain help, and a forum labeled "Technical Questions" should be provided. Student comments in this forum should be read and referred to appropriate resources or technical support team. The third type of forum is a content forum, which is used to discuss experiences with the course material. The fourth is a student lounge or a "coffee bar" which is used for non-course related discussions.

Discussion questions should be used to stimulate interaction among students and instructors. These questions should be open-ended and based on the relevant course content. These questions should stimulate student thinking and facilitate students learning from each other. For example, "How would you apply the principles from Unit 1 to your area of interest in nursing?" When done correctly, the answers to discussion questions will end in yet another question, thereby bringing the discussion to a higher level. For example, the student may end by saying, "Have others had a different experience?" Often it is necessary for the instructor to model this type of answer by offering their own experiences for the students to follow.

The guiding principles suggested by IDE (Innovations, undated) for Interaction are:

1. Interaction among learners should be frequent and meaningful and should occur between learners and instructional materials, and between learners and the instructor.
2. Participants should build confidence and competence with the learning process and supporting technologies.
3. Create and maintain learning communities for learners.
4. Use creative solutions to complete the objectives, to maintain interaction among faculty, students, and peers and to provide access to advising and academic support services and resources.
5. Encourage and support social interactions between and among learners.

A Course Design Model developed by Margaret Chambers (*http:// www.mindlinked.com*), Director of the Institute of Distance Education at the University of Maryland University College and the Web Initiative in Teaching Project instituted by the University System of Maryland from 1998 to 2002, outlines the following phases and components:

Phase One
Mapping: identify goals, issues and constraints
Architecture: reconceptualize the course and restructure into modules or educational objects
Prototype: design a sample-learning module illustrating the design decisions

Phase Two
Early Development: develop key elements, modules or educational objects for testing with students
Field Testing: critical elements with real students and colleagues
Late Development: complete courseware

Phase Three:
Institutional launch: arrange for course listing, marketing and registration: post a course review site
Pilot Course Delivery: teach the course online with external peer reviewers
Revision: modify and update

DEVELOPING A COURSE DESIGN

To facilitate the course design process, ALN (2000) suggests *The Yellow Sticky Method*. The steps in that process are as follows:

1. Gather pads of yellow stickies (post-it notes), a large piece of paper (or whiteboard) and a pen or marker.
2. On a sticky write "Homepage" and place it on the large piece of paper or whiteboard.
3. Consider your course platform, such as WebCT or Blackboard and write the key elements of your platform, each on a separate sticky, for example, syllabus, content (mental models), course material, communication, and assignments—and then organize them into a logical format on the large piece of paper or whiteboard.
4. Think how the course should be organized: the spread, the checklist, or the nodes? Move stickies around until you create the structure that makes most sense to you.
5. Use the pen or marker and draw lines to connect the pages and sections.
6. Focus on the "microlevel" — specific lectures and readings; create a sticky for each lecture, assignment, and quiz, and organize them on the board.
7. Consider learning strategies that you will use to disseminate the content.

ALN (2000) suggests a quality check: "Examine the pages you have created. Are all of the major features in place? Is there a clear and consistent navigational structure? Are your assignments, assessment criteria, and learning strategies in place and adequate for students to reach the course goals?" (p. 82).

IDE (Innovations, n.d.) also offers guiding principles for assessment and measurement and learner services and support, to be considered in designing online learning environments. The assessment and measurement principles are:

1. Assessment instruments and activities should be congruent with the learner's learning goals and skills.

2. Assessment and measurement strategies should enable the learner to assess their progress through the learning experience.
3. Assessment and measurement strategies should accommodate the special needs, characteristics, and situations of the learner.
4. Learners should have ample opportunities and accessible methods for providing feedback.

The guiding principles for learner services and support are:

1. A comprehensive system of technical support services should be in place to ensure the effective use of technologies in distance education programming for learners, instructors, and staff.
2. Faculty should have access to adequate support in instructional technology and distance education methodologies.
3. Support systems should be designed to provide service seven days a week, twenty-four hours a day for faculty and learners.
4. Regular feedback mechanisms should be designed and implemented to assess the successes and failures of the various support services.

SUMMARY

Design begins with an assessment of the learner and the technological expertise of the developer. Begin design with behavioral objectives that are appropriate to the learner and based on the content. The structure is dependent on the software platform but regardless of the "givens", multiple methods of learning should be included to accommodate various student learning styles. The learner can navigate via graphics or text but should be able to get where they want to go in three clicks (or less) of the mouse. The layout of every page should be identical and templated so the learner knows where they are and how to navigate to somewhere else. Learners need to communicate with each other and with the instructor. The most common form of communication is through bulletin boards, but there are other means of interacting through chat rooms and audio and video conferencing.

REFERENCES

ALN (2000). *Pre-conference workshop: Strategic planning for on-line courses*. ALN Conference at University of Maryland, University College, July, 2000.

Boshier, R., mohapi, M., Moulton, G., Qayyu, A., Sadownik, L.,Wilson, M. (1997). Best and worst dressed web courses: Strutting into the 21st century in comfort and style. *Distance Education, 18(2)*.

Brueckner, C.W. (1999). Seven steps to success designing online courses. Retrieved December 19, 2002 from *http://bass.sit.ecu.edu/FacultyResources/designingonline*.

Honebein, P.C. (1996). Seven goals for the design of constructivist learning environments. In B. Wilson, (Ed.). *Constructivist learning environments*. Englewood Clifts, NJ: Educational Technology Publications.

Illinois Online Network (ION). Retrieved October 17, 2002, from *http://illinois.online.uillinois.edu/IONresources/instructionalDesign/learningStyle.html*.

Innovations in Distance Education. Retrieved October 20, 2002, from *http://is124.ce.psu.edu/DE/IDE/guiding_principles/swsi/sum_by_cat.html*.

Learning to Learn: About Web-Based Instructional Design. Retrieved October 17, 2002, from http://snow.utoronto.ca/Learn2/design.html.

Reigeluth, C.M. (Ed.) (1999). *Instructional-design theories and models: A new paradigm of instructional theory. Volume II*. Mahwah, NJ: Lawrence Erlbaum Associates.

Smith, P.L. & Ragan, T.J. (1999). *Instructional design* (2nd ed.). New York: John Wiley & Sons.

Web Style Guide (2002). Retrieved October 1, 2003, from *http://www.webstyleguide.com/site/organize.html*.

Winn, W. (1991). A constructivist critique of the assumptions of instructional design. In T.M. Duffy (Ed),. *designing environments for constructive learning*. Berlin: Springer-Verlag.

Yale Style Manual. Retrieved October 18, 2002, from *http://info.med.yale.edu/caim/manual/sites/site_design.html*.

7

Course Management Methods

anaging an online course can have many similarities to
managing a face-to-face course but differs in complexity
with the use of technology and the geographic distance.
For example, setting the tone and establishing the setting are common to both situations. The role of the faculty, which requires
greater attention to detail, structure, and monitoring, will be different when establishing the online classroom. Facilitating learning at
a distance requires some new approaches to managing the teaching
and learning process. According to Kimball (2000), effective faculty
start with a completely new mindset about technology and must
learn to manage a new set of variables which determine the extent
to which their courses are effective. In this chapter, the role of the
instructor and the expectations of the student, along with planning,
organizing, and managing of online learning will be discussed.

FACULTY ROLE

The role of the instructor shifts from the traditional classroom
"sage on the stage" to the "guide on the side" instructor. Although
these might be overused phrases, there is a lot of truth to them as
they apply to the instructor role shift that takes place when teaching online. In a traditional setting, the instructor feeds information
to students in a lecture or PowerPoint slide presentation format.
This method of teaching has long been used in educational settings
and has come to be what most students expect. In a distance-

learning role, the instructor focuses on discussing and reviewing materials presented through video and/or audio technologies, assigned readings, and interactive group activities. The faculty role is that of content expert, who guides or facilitates student learning through direction to resources and stimulation of discussion.

Perhaps one of the most significant ways in which the faculty role changes is the way faculty develop courses, because courses often must be redesigned significantly to be compatible with, and maximize the use of, distance education delivery systems (Billings, 1997). According to the Illinois Online Network (n.d) "This brings new pressures on instructors, both to deal with a different way of teaching, interacting, and managing a 24–hour-a-day classroom populated by adults who demand relevance and may require extra support due to their already busy lives." Some responsibilities include:

- Planning and organizing the course
- Creating a collaborative atmosphere
- Constructing open-ended, thought-provoking questions
- Providing direction and leadership
- Setting the agenda
- Giving feedback and reinforcement
- Sequencing content and pacing the material

In order to perform these responsibilities, successful online faculty should have some basic background knowledge and preparation to teach online. According to ION (n.d.), the instructor should:

- Have a broad base of life experiences in addition to academic credentials in the subject matter. This will enable the instructor to actively participate with students and guide their constructive thinking.
- Be open, concerned, flexible, and sincere so they can compensate for the lack of physical presence.
- Feel comfortable communicating in writing because it is the basic element of the process.
- Believe that learning can occur in facilitated online learning environments.

- Believe that the online learning process includes learning information that can be used today and which requires critical thinking.
- Be supportive of the development of critical thinking.
- Have the appropriate credentials to teach the subject.
- Be well trained in teaching and learning online.

PLANNING AND ORGANIZING

When planning and organizing an online course, the instructor must look at the overall course in terms of objectives, outcomes, assessment, and evaluation. The planning should include the criteria discussed in the reconceptualization chapter 5 of this book. The instructor should keep in mind that it is in this beginning phase of course development that the expertise of an instructional designer and an information technology expert should be employed.

COLLABORATION

Once the course has been planned and organized, the instructor is ready to launch the course. It is now the instructor's responsibility to create a collaborative atmosphere. To create this environment, the students should encounter a warm and friendly welcoming message as they first enter your online course. This message could say something like, "Welcome! I'm going to be your instructor for this course. If you can read this message, then you have successfully joined our online classroom. Please check back frequently for further instructions, course materials, and discussions that will be relevant to your learning." Using an "ice breaker" such as requesting a short biography as the initial assignment will give students something to respond to. The instructor can post his or her bio first as an introduction and then ask the students to present theirs in a similar format. For example, the instructor can describe work experiences, educational background, course expectations, and some personal information. This is not only a way of introducing oneself to the class but also a way for the instructor to gain information about students that can be used later in class discussions. The students often find that they have similar backgrounds or professional interests, which then allows them to begin developing a sense of community through realization of shared goals and shared expectations of the course. By asking the learners to contribute their goals and expectations, the instructor is able to determine if the learners are all starting from the same place or if the instructor needs to shift her approach to correspond more closely to the needs of the learners.

Students should be encouraged to respond to each other's postings. The best way to teach students how to post meaningful statements is for the instructor to model how they should respond. Modeling a short but welcoming response does this best. Not only does this enable students to begin opening up to each other, but it begins creating a safe space in which they can interact. The posting of an introduction is the first step in revealing who one is to the others in the class and it is critical that they feel acknowledged so they can continue to do that safely throughout the duration of the course. This is the first point of connection—the point where these important relationships begin to develop (Palloff and Pratt, 1999).

DEVELOPING DISCUSSION QUESTIONS

Developing or creating open-ended questions is the primary method for stimulating discussion, assessing student learning and providing for interactivity amongst the learners. The discussion questions should be based on the desired learning outcomes and can vary in number based on instructor preference. Most faculty use approximately 2 to 4 discussion questions depending on the course schedule for the week. The discussion questions should be open-ended, thought provoking, but relevant to student learning. Then, the instructor as well as the students must learn the art of expansive questions in order to keep the discussion going. This allows the responsibility for facilitation of discussion to be shared among all participants. And finally, students should be encouraged to provide constructive feedback to one another throughout the course. Rather than being at the forefront of the discussion, the instructor is an equal player, acting as a gentle guide (Palloff & Pratt, 1999). The sharing of this responsibility among the participants is one way instructors can stretch their facilitative skills.

The discussion questions should be developed in a way that there is not a right or wrong answer. They serve to stimulate thinking and are a means by which the instructor can assess student learning and understanding of the issues. The instructor needs to model this form of questioning so that students can learn to answer questions in a substantive manner, provide an example, cite a resource, and end with an expansive question for his/her classmates. This allows for the discussion to progress to a higher level as questions are answered and expanded upon by students pursuing the issue. The instructor's role is to closely monitor the discussion and to jump in with another question, thereby expanding the level of thinking beyond the original question. A poor or minimal response to a question could indicate that student thinking has not been stimulated and that the learners have not been compelled or inspired to respond. Commenting on discussion questions by asking students for more information or by sharing some aspects of their professional expertise can help to engage students and facilitate online discussions.

DIRECTION AND LEADERSHIP

Providing direction and leadership in an online course should begin before the students enter the classroom. The syllabus or a separate document on how to run the course should be used to provide clear directions for students about:

- General information
- Contact information
- Textbooks or other course materials
- Course requirements
- Where to start
- How I plan to run this course
- Class schedule, parts of the classroom
- Group work and expectations

- Technical support
- Grading
- Student responsibility

General course information should include course start and end dates, and midterm and final exam dates. Also remember to include time off for spring break or other breaks related to holidays or official closing of the university. The University of Phoenix for example has a two-week winter break over the end-of-year holidays, which may fall in the middle of some classes. Contact information is important for students in order to have easy access to faculty. Often it is helpful to put a primary and a secondary e-mail address, work and home phone numbers (optional), and the best times to make contact. Times of contact are important especially when students are working shifts and faculty may be located in a different time zone.

Required texts and supporting documents should be available to students before class begins or at least during the first week of class. Students should have the ability to order books from either the bookstore or another online book service such as Amazon.com. Other recommended texts should be listed in case students are interested in purchasing these as well.

Course requirements help students know in advance what they will need to do and what faculty have identified as requirements to complete this course. For example, 1) View lecture material 2) Assigned readings 3) Team exercises 4) Assignments, 5) Midterm and final examination. Clearly listing requirements ahead of time will help students organize their approach to the course and will provide a high level view of course requirements.

"Where to Start" and "How I Plan to Run This Course" are opportunities to help students begin. Often in a face-to-face course this is the housekeeping session that takes place on the first day of class. When directing students where to start, it is critical to have students attend either a face-to-face or an online orientation. It is in this orientation that they will be instructed to obtain a password for the course and begin to learn basic navigation of the courseware if this is their first experience with online learning. Once students are inside the online course, they should be directed to read the course information carefully. This should include the syllabus and all supporting documents that will be used to run the course. "How I plan to run this course" can include an explanation such as this:

> As you may have gathered by now, taking an online course is NOT an easy way out. It requires every bit as much time (if not more) than a face-to-face course. You must be self-directed and must keep up with the class in order to know what is going on, what is taking place in the main classroom, what are the answers to the questions being asked, when the assignments are due, and so on. I expect you to log in at least 3–4 times a week in addition to the time you will spend doing readings and project assignments. My plan is to be online every day for the first couple of weeks until we get going and then 3–4 times a week once things are underway. I expect you to check in to the course about the same number of times to check the Announcements and to begin interacting in the course.

The idea is to let students know what will be done to run the course and then to have them follow that lead.

The course schedule can be placed in a calendar and should include important dates that students should note. (See Table 7.1) For example, weekly lectures and discussion questions will be posted every Monday. Discussion question answers should be posted by Wednesday; Weekly summary should be posted by Friday. This schedule will help students develop some structure for their learning and help them to juggle their workload. Let them know when quizzes will be posted, and again take the opportunity to highlight due dates of midterms, final exams, and papers. One lesson for faculty that cannot be overstated is that *you cannot be too redundant in the online environment.* The more places a student can find important dates, the better. The main parts of the classroom should also be clearly delineated. If using courseware such as Blackboard or WebCT, the left menu bar is a good place to start. For example:

> **Announcements:** You will be on the Announcements page when you sign in. This is very important for you to watch frequently. I will post important reminders for you on this page regarding quizzes, assignments and tests.
>
> **Course Information:** This section contains many documents that will be

useful for you in this course. Like this one for example! Also your syllabus, course packet, quizzes, sample APA formatted paper, instructions on submitting assignements and more.

Faculty Information: This section contains my contact information (as above) as well as other contact information that might be useful to you while enrolled in this course.

Assignments: This section contains the instructions for the individual assignments for this course and the grading criteria.

Course Documents: This is where you will find the lectures for this course. Additionally, the objectives, readings, and supplemental Web links for each lecture can also be found here.This is the primary location for the course content.

Student Tools: This is where you will find the digital drop box, student grades, calendar, and other tools. Your grades are only available to you (and the instructor) because each student's course is protected by their own password. You will need to know how to use the digital drop box when you turn in assignments. I will post instructions for you (state where?). Check course information!

By identifying the parts of the online classroom, orientation information is restated and a text document is provided for reference (see Table 7.1). Once this document is written, it is highly reusable except for dates or changes that have taken place in the course. Technical support contact information should also be provided in the form of hours of availability, phone numbers and e-mail. Although this information is provided, invariably technical questions will show up in the discussion area of the classroom. Posting a message thread for technical questions will often allow students to answer each other's questions and keep the questions separate from the course content of the main classroom.

Grading information should also be clearly delineated in terms of: 1) methods of evaluation (i.e., class exercises, assignments, papers, and exams), and 2) criteria for the final grade. For example:

Participation	10%
Team Exercises	30%
Midterm Exam	30%
Final Exam	30%
Total	100%

Just as in face-to-face classes, students need to know the weight of graded assignments. They should also know what numerical value is required for an A, B, etc. This is also a good place to include the policy on late assignments (regarding point reduction) or incomplete grades, and information about the university's policy on academic integrity.

One aspect of ensuring quality and academic integrity is finding ways to document student identity as related to course assignments and testing. In short, faculty need to be sure that individuals receiving course credit are, indeed, the individuals who do the work (Tulloch & Thompson, 1999). There are a variety of ways to achieve identity security in the context of a meaningful assessment. The choices that an institution has will depend on the institutional resources, the type of assessment appropriate for measuring achievement of the learning objectives, and the number of students that need to be served. While high-tech methodologies exist for secure identification, such as retinal scanning or facial, voice, or fingerprint identification, institutions may not be ready to invest in these technologies. Another alternative is proctored testing centers or Web-based testing software. This software requires a user name and password and can provide a different test each time the user logs in.

SETTING THE AGENDA

The course agenda includes the nonnegotiable parts of the course (i.e., those that cannot be changed). The course agenda allows the student to anticipate what to expect from the course in terms of an overall preview. On a more detailed level, an agenda should provide students with information about what to expect on a weekly basis. The overall course agenda could be incorporated into the syllabus and the course calendar and could include information such as objectives, due dates of assignments, midterms, and finals. The overall agenda will allow students to organize their time around important dates and course deliverables. The weekly agenda will allow students to organize their week. For example, at the beginning of every week the instructor could post the weekly objectives, the reading assignments, and the individual and group assignments. By having these agenda items available and even at times redundant, the students will be more unlikely to miss important information that is necessary for course completion. Do not hesitate to repeat instructions and post assignment reminders of deadlines, as this can be very helpful for students.

SEQUENCE AND PACE

The sequence and pace of providing lectures and assignments can be left to the instructor's discretion. Some instructors prefer to post lectures, assignments, and discussion questions on a week-by-week basis. This controls the pace of the course and does not allow the students to work ahead. This model would most closely replicate the sequence and pace of a face-to-face classroom. Some instructors like to guide the online classroom discussion using this strategy. Another option would be to release course content by units, clusters, or modules. For example, in an online informatics course, the instructor may choose to post quarterly based on clusters of course information. The lecture for the electronic health record, the electronic health record system, and data mining could all be posted simultaneously which then allows the students to work ahead if they choose. Using this strategy, the instructor would still want to control the discussion by posting discussion questions regularly within the block of time designated for a particular unit. A third strategy for sequencing the release of course content would be to give the student the entire course at the beginning of class. Some instructors may not even have the entire course ready at the beginning of the course or may use the early weeks of a course to do revisions. The University of Phoenix Online, for example, provides the students with a course module that is the entire course, but the students are required to participate according to the instructor's instructions. The instructor will post a weekly lecture, assignment, and discussion questions, and the student is expected to keep pace with the instructor's lead. This strategy allows students to work ahead in their reading, writing, and group work but also allows the instructor to control the collaborative learning in the main discussion area of the classroom. Some instructors have found it useful to put start and stop dates on discussions. For example, if a particular discussion thread is only going to be open for two weeks, the instructor should post start and stop dates at the beginning of the message thread so that students know when to move on to the next topic.

FEEDBACK

Feedback is one of the most critical activities that instructors need to be aware of in online learning because of the lack of face-to-face interaction. Feedback goes beyond confirmation of correct answers. Feedback is necessary for students to develop new understandings and to facilitate learning (Perrin, 1999). It is necessary for instructors to respond to students in a timely manner (usually within 24–48 hours) in order for students to not feel that they are being ignored. Online students need extra reinforcement and verification of their performance. Positive feedback, constructive feedback, and tone are all areas that instructors need to be aware of and sensitive to when responding to students. For example, proposing an alternative viewpoint might be interpreted by a student as an incorrect statement on his/her part as opposed to just an expansion of ideas. Without hearing the tone in which feedback was given, a student could easily sit there and wonder, "Did I say something wrong?" Without really knowing how a remark was interpreted, the student may decide not to ask or decide not to speak up in the future. While maintaining a positive and encouraging tone and keeping things light with humor and emoticons, the instructor can still maintain a professional atmosphere in the class environment.

It is known that communicating with students and influencing their learning positively is done on the basis of feedback. "The National Report on Learning," published by the U.S. Department of Education in the 1980s stressed that improvement in learning is more likely to occur following both written and oral critiques of student work. Therefore it should be a significant approach to improve grading by providing more information than solely a number or letter symbol on an assignment. Oral critiques can be provided by telephone to students, but more likely will occur by e-mail. The following characteristics should be considered in providing personal feedback to students:

- multidimensional — covers content, presentation, and grammar
- Nonevaluative (provides objective information)
- Supportive (offers information that will allow the learner to see areas for improvement)
- Receiver Controlled (allows the learner to accept or reject the information)
- Timely (provided as soon as possible after the intended work)
- Specific (precisely describes observations and recommendations)

The instructor should be sure to provide information at the beginning of class so that students know what is expected of them and what will be standard for evaluation and feedback. Instructor feedback should be clear, thorough, consistent, equitable, and professional. Since students require regular and constructive feedback from faculty, they will appreciate comments that indicate the instructor has tailored remarks for that particular individual.

NETIQUETTE

Netiquette, or Internet etiquette are guidelines for posting and sending messages in the online classroom. Netiquette not only covers rules of behavior but also guidelines for ensuring interaction in the online environment. Shea (1999) outlined core rules of netiquette that every online student should follow:

- Remember the human (never forget there is really a person)
- Adhere to the same standards of behavior online that you follow in real life (in other words, be ethical)
- Know when you are in cyberspace (i.e. main discussion area, chat area)

- Respect each other's time and bandwidth (post appropriate messages)
- Make yourself look good online (check grammar and spelling)
- Share expert knowledge (help answer others' questions)
- Help keep tempers under control (don't respond to irate postings)
- Respect other people's privacy (do not read others private e-mail)
- Don't abuse your power
- Be forgiving of other people's mistakes (you were once new to the online environment as well).

The core rules of netiquette were designed to help students who are new to the Internet to make friends instead of enemies. The instructor can post these basic rules to help students understand the basic expectations of behavior online.

SPECIAL CONSIDERATIONS

Diversity and Americans with disabilities, are global issues facing us daily as well as in the online environment. Since these issues are considered serious and sensitive to many people, instructors should consider human equity issues seriously.

Key Points on Diversity

Diversity consists of two dimensions, primary and secondary.

- Primary dimensions are those characteristics that everyone is born with and that are visible and easy to identify. They include age, gender, race, ethnicity, and other physical characteristics.
- Secondary dimensions are differences or characteristics that we acquire or change throughout our lives. These include work experience, income, marital status, religious beliefs, and education. These dimensions shape everyone we en-

counter in school, the workplace, and social settings. Valuing diversity according to the Center for Research on Education, Diversity and Excellence (2002) is:

- Voluntary
- Productivity driven
- Qualitative
- Opportunity focused
- Proactive

Government, corporation, and educational institutions are now recognizing the necessity of valuing diversity to remain competitive and effective. As a facilitator, one needs to eliminate stereotypes and become more educated about different groups. This way one is less likely to generalize. Suggestions for doing this might include:

- becoming aware of the stereotypes you hold
- determining the source of the stereotype and how it was formed
- expanding your knowledge about other groups/cultures
- expanding your experiences with other groups/cultures

Key points of American with Disabilities Act

The Americans with Disabilities Act, 42 U.S.C. secs. 12101, et seq., directs universities to make their distance learning classes accessible to qualified individuals with a disability, just as they are required to do for traditional courses. In particular, 42 U.S.C. sec. 12132 states:

Subject to the provisions of this subchapter, no qualified individual with a disability shall, by reason of such disability, be excluded from participation in or be denied the benefits of the services, programs, or activities of a public entity, or be subjected to discrimination by any such entity.

For nonpublic institutions, 42 U.S.C. sec. 12182(a) provides:

No individual shall be discriminated against on the basis of disability in the full and equal enjoyment of the goods, services, facilities, privileges, advantages, or accommodations of any place of public accommodation by any person who owns, leases (or leases to), or operates a place of public accommodation.

As universities and faculty expand their distance-education offerings, they are finding that they must include the virtual equivalents of wheelchair ramps when building their online classrooms. They must accommodate, for instance, the student who is unable to see navigational graphics on a Web page because he's blind, and the student who can't listen to a streaming audio lecture because she's deaf. In fact, many students with disabilities find that Web site technological extravaganzas are more of a burden than an aid.

For the most part, distance-education students with disabilities already can get the equipment they need to make up for their impairments. Blind students can use software that reads online text aloud or produces a Braille message for the students to follow. Students who cannot move their arms easily can use adaptive equipment to manipulate the computer with other parts of their bodies. But some common features of the Internet make navigation difficult for people with certain disabilities. Text-reading programs, for instance, are unable to recognize graphics. The problem is easily avoided if the programs can pick up and read aloud alternate texts that are placed behind the graphics, but not every Web site provides those texts. Sites with frames and tables (two commonly used features of Web-page design) tend to confuse those programs, which often read from left to right, ignoring the layout. An important issue is for universities to determine exactly what the law requires.

The California Community Colleges System has a published set of tips for online faculty: Provide clear, prominent navigation mechanisms (for those who can't click on small links). And don't rely on color alone to distinguish characteristics of a page (for students who are color blind). The goal is for virtual classrooms to be held to the same accessibility standards as conventional classrooms. Several online services also help Website designers build accessible pages. A program called "Bobby" checks pages and points out potential problems of access (*http://www.cast.org/bobby/*). The program was created by the Center for Applied Special Technology, an organization devoted to using technology to expand opportunities for everyone, including people with disabilities.

As an online facilitator, the considerations for students with disabilities need to be taken on an individual basis. For example, if you know a student has a particular disability, you will need to take into account accommodations that may be necessary for this particular problem. It should be determined from the beginning exactly what the student's limitations are and what devices the student is using, if any, for example, TTY phones, screen readers, or voice recognition software. Allowing more time for test taking may be necessary for some individuals, or allowance for leniency on spelling if you know a student is using voice recognition software. If you are using audio files for example, be sure to include a text version of the same information. If you are including Web references, be sure to check their format (amount of graphics, use of frames) for accommodating screen readers. *The bottom line is that everyone should have equal access to information.*

STUDENT ROLE

The student role in a distance course also changes significantly. Students must be more responsible for their own learning and there is greater emphasis on identifying one's own learning needs and making plans to achieve learning objectives (Billings, 1997). Prior to becoming an online student, the individual must have some basic knowledge of information technology in order to participate in a distance course. Gilbert (2001) suggests that students start by asking:

- What is online learning and what is it like?
- Where can I find it and is it for me?
- What works in an online environment?
- What criteria make a good candidate for online learning?
- What are the advantages or disadvantages?
- How do I choose an online learning provider?
- How do I pick a curriculum?
- How can I get information about sources?

- What makes for a good distance program
- Where do I start?
- How can I succeed?
- How can I manage the tools and equipment?

When designing distance learning academic programs, the basic characteristics of students should be considered. Their age, interests, skill levels, academic preparedness, and career goals, for example should be considered. Much of the literature suggests that older students and adults are the primary targets of distance programs. In the United States, typical adult distance learning students are between the ages of twenty-five and fifty. Many online learners are adult students with family and job responsibilities who require the flexibility of online learning in order to advance in their job or to earn their degree. However, as more and more younger and older people become aware of the online learning model, the traditional profile is changing.

So what criteria should the online student consider when doing a self-evaluation for distance learning? The Illinois Online Network (2001) suggests that the student possess the following qualities:

- *Be open minded about sharing life, work, and educational experiences as part of the learning process.* Introverts as well as extroverts find that the online process requires them to utilize their experiences. This forum for communication eliminates the visual barriers that hinder some individuals in expressing themselves. In addition, the student is given time to reflect on the information before responding. The online environment should be open and friendly.
- *Be able to communicate through writing.* In the Virtual Classroom, nearly all communication is written, so it is critical that students feel comfortable in expressing themselves in writing. Many students have limited writing abilities, which should be addressed before or as part of the online experience. This may require remedial efforts on the part of the student.
- *Be self-motivated and self-disciplined.* With the freedom and flexibility of the online environment comes responsibility.

The online process takes a real commitment and discipline to keep up with the flow of the process.

- *Be willing to "speak up" if problems arise.* Many of the nonverbal communication mechanisms that instructors use in determining whether students are having problems (confusion, frustration, boredom, absence, etc.) are not possible in the online paradigm. If a student is experiencing difficulty on any level (either with the technology or with the course content), he or she must communicate this immediately. Otherwise the instructor will never know what is wrong.

- *Be willing and able to commit to 4 to 15 hours per week per course.* Online is not easier than the traditional educational process. In fact, many students will say it requires much more time and commitment.

- *Be able to meet the minimum requirements for the program.* The requirements for online are no less than that of any other quality educational program. The successful student will view online as a convenient way to receive their education—not an easier way.

- *Accept critical thinking and decision making as part of the learning process.* The learning process requires the student to make decisions based on facts as well as experience. Assimilating information and executing the right decisions requires critical thought; case analysis does this very effectively.

- *Have access to a computer and a modem.* The communication medium is a computer, phone line, and modem; the student must have access to the necessary equipment.

- *Be able to think ideas through before responding.* Meaningful and quality input into the virtual classroom is an essential part of the learning process. Time is given in the process to allow for the careful consideration of responses. The testing and challenging of ideas is encouraged; you will not always be right, just be prepared to accept a challenge.

- *Feel that high quality learning can take place without going to a traditional classroom.* If the student feels that a traditional classroom is a prerequisite to learning, they may be more comfortable in the traditional classroom. Online is not for everybody. A student who wants to be on a traditional campus attending a traditional classroom is probably not going to be happy online. While the level of social interaction can be very high in the virtual classroom, it is not the same as living in a dorm on a campus. This should be made known. An online student is expected to:

· Participate in the virtual classroom 3–5 out of 7 days a week
· Be able to work with others in completing projects
· Be able to use the technology properly
· Be able to meet the minimum standards as set forth by the institution
· Be able to complete assignments on time
· Enjoy communicating in writing. In your online course, you may want to include reference links to resources and tips for your students to use to help them be more successful online learners. Many universities have information on their home page that helps students with tips for success in online courses. Clearly outlining expectations and characteristics of a successful online student can help students determine if the online environment will be a productive learning environment for them. Often a questionnaire for prospective students to fill out to assess whether they are good candidates for online learning can be found on the university home page.

STUDENT EXPECTATIONS

Online students should expect that their instructor would provide the best learning environment possible. According to ION (2001) the student should expect that:

- The instructor will create the learning environment in such a way that learners can use their own experiences in the learning process and to translate theory to practice
- The instructor should be concerned about the success of the learner and every reasonable opportunity should be given to the learner to achieve
- The instructor should give and solicit feedback. The feed-

back given by the instructor should keep the learner aware of their progress in the course. The feedback the instructor elicits from learners should guide the students progress toward attaining objectives
- The student should expect little or no lecturing
- Tests that require memorization are least effective and case analysis would be more appropriate
- The learner will be treated politely and respectfully
- The instructor should be online everyday, or at least 5 times a week

With consistency in instructor delivery, students can anticipate and prepare their coursework based on expectations of how the instructor will run the course. When managing an online course, the faculty and the student play important roles. The faculty must plan for how the course will be managed based on student profiles, and the student must take responsibility for learning. A variety of characteristics including demographics, motivation, academic preparedness, and access to resources should be considered as important for an online learner.

SUMMARY

Course management covers a breadth of considerations from student orientation to discussion facilitation to instructor feedback for students. It is interesting to note that each time an online course is taught, the instructor will note nuances or frequently asked questions that will help to prepare better for the next time the class is taught. The students eventually will come armed with experience of online learning and will focus less on technology and management issues and more on course content.

REFERENCES

Billings, D. (1997). Issues in teaching and learning at a distance: Changing roles and responsibilities of administrators, faculty and students. *Computers in Nursing* 15(2); 69–70.

Center for Research on Education, Diversity and Excellence (2002). Retrieved January 23, 2003, from *http://www.crede.ucsc.edu*.

Gilbert, S. (1999). *How to be a successful online student*. New York: McGraw-Hill.

Kimball, L. (1998). Managing distance learning—new challenges for faculty. In the Digital university Springer, London.

Palloff R. & Pratt K. (1999). *Building learning communities in cyberspace; Effective strategies for the online classroom*. San Francisco: Jossey-Bass Publishers.

Perrin, D. (1999). The level of interactivity on the internet and the web. Retrieved January 20, 1999, from *http://usdla.org/html/journal/APR99_Issue/16_ed_apr_99c.htm*.

Shea, V. (1999). Net Etiquette. Retrieved January 15, 2003, from *http://www.albion.com/netiquette/introduction.html*.

Tulloch, J., & Thompson, S. (1999). Identity security and testing issues in distance learning: The Agenda. Retrieved June 20, 2003 from *http://www.pbs.org/als/agenda/articles/testing.html*.

Illinois Learning Network (2001). Retrieved January 15, 2003, from *http://www.ion.illinois.edu/IONresources/onlineLearning/StudentProfile.html*.

TABLE 7.1 Sample of an Online Syllabus

Please print a copy of this document for handy reference

UNIVERSITY OF xxxxxxx
COURSE SYLLABUS
COURSE NUMBER: xxxxxxxx
COURSE TITLE: Nursing 301
COURSE START DATE: xxxxxx
COURSE END DATE: xxxxxx
INSTRUCTOR—Your Name
Email Address: xxxxxxxHome Telephone Number: xxxxxxxx Eastern Standard Time
Alternative/emergency e-mail address: xxxxxxx
Instructor Availability: Indicate the best times and methods for students to reach you here.
Welcome class!
Provide a welcoming message and a brief bio on yourself.

GENERAL COURSE DESCRIPTION

This course develops the basic skills of critically analyzing research findings. Research methods are introduced with emphasis placed upon analyzing key elements of research reports.

TOPICS AND OBJECTIVES

Provide a course overview here.

CLASS BIOGRAPHIES—Your first assignment is to post a biography in the main classroom using mine as a suggested format. Please feel free to use the chat area to respond to each other's bios and informally get to know each other.

Student materials

BOOKS, SOFTWARE, OR OTHER COURSE MATERIALS
List books required for the course here and a link to the university library

ELECTRONIC RESOURCES
Provide relevant course links here.

WHERE TO GO TO CLASS—YOUR CLASS MEETINGS

COMMUNICATION: This is the *MAIN* discussion area for the class. It has access for everyone. This is our *main classroom*.

ASSIGNMENTS can be submitted to the digital drop box or to the instructors email.

CHAT ROOM is designed as a place to discuss issues not related to the course content, but you can use it for discussion questions and things like that if you want.

COURSEMATERIALS provide relevant documents for completing this course

GROUP WORK :

Learning-Team A
Learning-Team B
Learning-Team C
Learning-Team D

TECHNOLOGY ISSUES:
For problems with access into this course or other technology issues, please contact the university help desk or other designated location for online courses. Email: xxxxxx Phone Numer: xxxxxx

APA AND ATTACHMENTS:
Some of your assignments require APA format. It is not possible to apply all the APA guidelines and have them transfer properly in OE notes, and so the University now requires that any assignments requiring APA format must be sent as attachments.

- Prepare these assignments in Microsoft Word
- Save your work as a ".doc" file (this is the MS Word default file type).
- To send an attachment, open a "Reply Group" in the correct thread (or a new post if it is to the Assignments folder)
- Type in a subject line that includes the name of the assignment and your initials
- Use the "Attach" function to find and attach the file from your word processor.
- Then send it.

THE ONLINE WEEKLY SCHEDULE: Please take note of the electronic weekly schedule. Remember that the week begins on Monday and ends on Sunday.
Day 1—Monday
Day 2—Tuesday
Day 3—Wednesday
Day 4—Thursday
Day 5—Friday
Day 6—Saturday
Day 7—Sunday

ADMINISTRATIVE ISSUES
COURSE CHANGES—Although I will not make changes in the objectives of the course or change the course materials, I reserve the right to make slight modifications of the weekly assignments that vary from the curriculum as necessary

ATTENDANCE—In order to meet the university requirements for attendance, you must post at least one message to the course discussion board on two separate days during the online week. If you are out of attendance for one week or more of a class that is four weeks in length, or two or more weeks of a course that is five or more weeks, you will be automatically withdrawn and not be eligible to receive credit or earn a credit grade. (Please note: Check your university's policy on attendance)

PARTICIPATION—Class participation is different from attendance. I expect each student to contribute to the class in a substantive way on X out of seven days each week. By substantive, I mean postings that demonstrate thought and an attempt to discuss your personal work experiences, as they are relevant to the class discussion (approximately 100–150 words). I will **not** be counting participation in the study group area as class participation. Please remember that I am looking for quality, not necessarily quantity.

LATE ASSIGNMENTS—Late assignments will be downgraded by one point for each day that they are late. An assignment is considered late if it is posted after midnight your time zone on the day it is due. If unforeseen circumstances prohibit you from turning in an assignment on time, be sure to contact me to negotiate for an alternative submission date.

WRITING ASSIGNMENTS—All papers must adhere to the university writing style guidelines. (Little, Brown Compact Handbook or APA Manual) Written assignments must include a cover page, abstract, and references. Your written work is a representation of you. Insure all credits are given for other's work. Any violations, plagiarism, or copying will not be tolerated. * *Please also ensure all written assignments have a defined summary at the end of the paper.*

INCOMPLETE GRADES—I do not grant "incompletes" in my class. Therefore it is imperative that you submit all final graded requirements by their due date.

WEEKLY SUMMARY—Each week you will present a brief (250 words or less) weekly summary that summarizes what you learned from the readings, research, activities, and assignments. This summary is due at the end of each week. Please include two paragraphs summarizing 1) what you learned from the course materials and 2) what you learned from your classmates. Students are not expected to present a weekly summary for the final week of the course.

GROUP WORK—Learning teams (or groups) will be developed on Sunday during the first week of class. You will be asked to participate in **one** of these groups (group A, B, or C) I will be assigning you to a group based on backgrounds and experience. GROUP WORK—you will receive your first group assignment on xxxxx. You will then work with this group for the remainder of the course. Your grade for your group work will be the same for all group members. Your group project *final* postings will be in the MAIN Classroom so that you can share your final product with your classmates. Please feel free to contact me if you feel strongly about working with a particular individual in your group or if any problems arise. (Some people prefer to work together by time zones or work schedules). Just remember, all work is asynchronous so we should accommodate everyone!

ACADEMIC HONESTY
Academic honesty is highly valued at online just as it is at each University setting. A student must always submit work that represents his or her original words or ideas. If any words or ideas are used that do not represent the student's original words or ideas, the student must cite all relevant sources. The student should also make clear the extent to which such sources were used. Words or ideas that require citations include, but are not limited to, all hard copy or electronic publications, whether copyrighted or not, and all verbal or visual communication when the content of such communication clearly originates from an identifiable source. At the online campus, all submissions to any public meeting or private mailbox fall within the scope of words and ideas that require citations if used by someone other than the original author.

Academic dishonesty in an online learning environment could involve:

- Having a tutor or friend complete a portion of your assignments
- Having a reviewer make extensive revisions to an assignment
- Copying work submitted by another student to a public class meeting
- Using information from online information services without proper citation.

GRADING FORMULA—I will not round grades numerically (either up or down) when it comes to graded papers and projects. I will not round on final grades. For example, final grade of 89.9 will be considered a B; however, other factors such as the quality of your participation will be considered.

Your overall class participation grade is based upon your general comments and interactions in all the forums, your Discussion Question inputs to the Main Forum, and your weekly overviews. You will get a chance to submit your own answers to the Discussion Questions as well as selectively comment on the submissions ofinterest made by other students. I will assign a participation grade each week (based on your general comments and overall interactions). Your Discussion Question responses are worth 5%, the timeliness and quality of your comments to other student Discussion Question responses are worth 5%, and your weekly overviews are worth 5%. The average for these grades will equal 15% of your final grade. I will give you weekly feedback using points to let you know how you are doing. For example, if you provide great answers to the discussion questions, participate actively and thoughtfully in the discussions and demonstrate what you have learned in your weekly summary, then you will have earned your full 3 points for the week!!

GRADING

94–100 = A
90–93 = A-
87–89 = B+
83–86 = B

80–82 = B-
77–79 = C+
73–76 = C
70–72 = C-
67–69 = D+
63–66 = D
60–62 = D-

POINT VALUES FOR THE COURSE ASSIGNMENTS

ASSIGNMENTS	*Percent*
Individual (70%)	
Paper One (Due end of week One)	10
Paper Two (Due end of week Two)	10
Paper Three (Due end of week Three)	10
Paper Four (Due end of week Four)	15
Paper Five (Due end of week Five)	15
Participation (Weekly)	10
Learning Team (30%)	
Presentation One (Due end of week Four)	15
Presentation Two (Due end of week Five)	15
Total	**100**

COURSE SCHEDULE

WEEK 1
Objectives:
  Readings

  Assignments

  Group Assignments

WEEK 2
Objectives:
  Readings

Assignments

Group Assignments

WEEK 3
Objectives:
Readings

Assignments

Group Assignments

WEEK 4
Objectives:
Readings

Assignments

Group Assignments

Week 5
Objectives:
Readings

Assignments

Group Assignments

**Please let me know if you find errors in this document. Thank you.
* **End of syllabus** *

8

Interacting and Communicating Online

Instructional interactivity takes place among the instructor, the learners and the content (Figure 8.1) and with each interaction is important for instructional design. In a traditional classroom, communication between the teacher and student and between students is generally synchronous (occurring at the same time and place). In distance learning, communication can be synchronous or asynchronous (not occurring at the same time). This chapter will discuss different types of interaction and communication that are well-suited for distance courses.

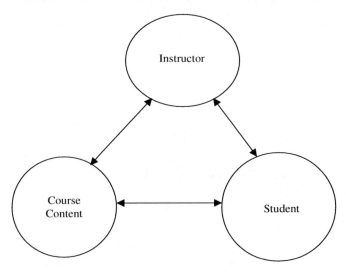

FIGURE 8.1 Elements of interaction in online learning environments.

IMPORTANCE OF INTERACTION

A successful online course is easy to access, easy to navigate, and interactive. Interactivity, however, means more than just clicking a mouse to advance to the next page. Interactivity requires meaningful feedback (fi.e., leading toward an established goal) for each learner. Often this involves written confirmation of a correct response, or a dialog with the instructor or other learners. In the online environment, interaction can take place in the form of a question and answer, an essay, or a discussion, and may be asynchronous or synchronous.

Characteristics of a "good" online conversation, according to Sherry, Travalin, and Billig (2000), include evidence of problem-solving, informed decision making, and depth of both student and teacher facilitated discussions. There should also be evidence of episodes that extend the conversation beyond a simple question/answer interaction to the examination of complex problems from multiple perspectives. For example, if a discussion were started on the topic of bioterrorism, the facilitator should try to elicit comments from an acute care and a community health nursing perspective. The questions should be open-ended and force students to hypothesize and develop their own questions on the subject.

ASYNCHRONOUS COMMUNICATION: INSTRUCTOR TO STUDENT

As stated above, asynchronous communication occurs at different times. It is characterized by time-independence meaning that the sender and receiver communicate with time delays. When preparing online courses, instructors build into the instructional design mechanisms for instructor to student interaction and communication from an asynchronous perspective.

Asynchronous communication uses the Internet for e-mail, electronic bulletin board, or web-based software. E-mail allows for personal and, therefore, private communication. The electronic bulletin board is used for a group e-mail or mailing list that allows all participants to post and read messages. This form of asynchronous communication is most commonly used in main discussion areas of online classrooms and allows students to interact with faculty, other students, and course content.

Instructor and student interaction with course content comprise a critical element of learning according to Picciano (2001). In traditional environments, textbooks, notes written on chalkboards, diagrams shown on overhead projectors, slide shows and video clips comprise the instructional content for a class (Picciano, 2001). In distance courses instructors can decide how best to deliver course content along with the guidance of an instructional designer. The University of Phoenix Online, for example, offers nursing lectures with guidelines for development of text-based instruction. The idea behind this simplified delivery mode is that a minimal amount of bandwidth is required for students to access course content. More sophisticated delivery modes include Power Point slides (with or without voice synchronization), flash presentations and streaming video. However, the instructor should not convert materials used in traditional courses without considering how distance technologies can allow the course materials to be used more effectively and efficiently. Additionally, the instructor needs to consider whether the students are able to access multimedia requiring plugins for viewing and access to large data files. Since many students still access the Internet using dial-up modems, the time required to download large files should be supplemented with a smaller file option (i.e., a text version of an audio file). This way the students will have options for accessing course information based on preference and hardware capability.

Depending on how the technology is used, distance learning content may be easier for students to use or interact with than traditional classroom content. Instructor notes or slides available for print from the course site allow students to take notes more thoroughly while listening to online lectures.

Graphics and or animated images available online can be viewed over and over by students without having to go to the library or nursing lab. Animated graphics create simulations to demonstrate blood flow or actions of the cranial nerves helping students to visualize body processes better than a one-dimensional textbook is capable of showing.

STUDENT TO STUDENT INTERACTIONS

Student to student interaction using asynchronous communication can take place in the main discussion area of an online course or in collaborative groups. The main discussion area of an online course should be analogous to the main classroom in a face-to-face course. This discussion area is where the students and instructor should meet to participate in active dialogue and discuss course material. It is also where students have the opportunity to learn from each other and ask questions for further understanding of course content. It is exactly this interaction that is an important component of the learning dynamic according to Picciano (2001). Technology is responsible for bringing students together, and because it takes some extra effort, the result is actually more interaction (Gilbert, 2001). Since students are not anonymous especially when drawn in by the instructor, the result is active participation that is often not observed in a face-to-face classroom. Students often feel less inhibited and have time to collect their thoughts prior to speaking up in an asynchronous discussion.

GROUP COLLABORATION

Groups or learning teams are another means by which the instructor can promote collaboration and interaction in the online classroom. Creating teams is useful for the purpose of small group discussion, completion of group assignments, engagement in small group activities, and simulations (Palloff & Pratt, 1999). Teams can be formed by offering students the opportunity to self-select membership or by instructor assignment. Sometimes students like to work together based on past experience and sometimes by time zones. Once groups are formed, it is important to post guidelines and expectations of team performance. For example:

1. Each team will designate/elect/appoint a team coordinator/ leader.
2. The leader will remain the same throughout the course unless replaced by a majority vote of the team or by the instructor.

3. The team leader may make a decision unless overruled by a majority.
4. Any project assigned to the team will receive a grade that applies to every member of that group.
5. The team leader will have the final authority to modify any team member's grade up or down (except for his/her own).
6. The instructor will have the final say in all cases where the team cannot reach a decision.

Within these guidelines it is expected that the team members will evaluate each other's work, participate, and contribute to the team assignment. Team self-evaluation is an option to offer teams to help promote a productive work environment.

SYNCHRONOUS COMMUNICATION

Synchronous communication can take place in the form of live chat rooms, or interactive video conferencing. The greatest challenge faced with synchronous communication or meetings is to coordinate a time in which all participants are available. Considerations that need to be made are differences in time zones and nurses working different shifts. Students often request that a live chat section of the course be available because it reduces feelings of isolation. However, it is rarely a productive discussion and frequently disintegrates into simple one-line contributions of minimal depth. Palloff and Pratt (1999) describe how chat sessions can replicate face-to-face classroom discussion, but in fact it is probably the fastest typist who will contribute the greatest amount to the discussion. Additionally, synchronous discussion can rapidly get out of sync because if a slower typist responds to a comment after several other points have been made, the responses no longer follow in order. Guidelines for participation should be established from the start so that the students have clear expectations of how the chat room will work. Some instructors prefer to use the synchronous chat feature of the classroom for office hours only. This gives the student the opportunity to interact with the instructor in real time and have any pertinent questions answered immediately.

The logistics of timing a live chat meeting can truly be reason enough not to use them. If students are working shifts in different time zones, it may be impossible to find a time that is convenient for all. Nurses working the night shift may have to get up in the middle of the day to participate. This will lead to reduced quality in their contributions and disruption in sleep prior to going back to work. When students are dispersed internationally, the window for meeting times is again reduced.

In the online environment, net meetings using Web cameras can take place but this technology currently works best for small numbers of individuals. Synchronous video conferencing requires students to be at a certain place at a certain time and is not yet advanced enough to be used in online courses. Possibilities for actual participation in lectures offered in remote places exist, but may require that the student visit a campus that has the video conferencing technology in place. This technology allows students in several locations to share the same learning experience simultaneously through two-way video and audio.

BUILDING COMMUNITY

Regardless of whether you use asynchronous or synchronous communication in the online classroom, the students should be helpful to feel as if they are a part of the learning community from the start. Distance students often feel isolated and alone in their early experiences online, but with proper guidance and personalized attention they quickly bond and come to depend on each other for learning and moral support. It is the instructors' responsibility for facilitating the personal and social aspects of an online community in order to create a successful learning experience (Palloff & Pratt, 1999). Collins and Berge (1996) discuss promoting human relationships by affirming and recognizing students' input, providing opportunities for students to develop a sense of group cohesiveness, maintaining the group as a unit, and helping members to work together in a mutual cause as necessary elements for building community in an online environment.

So how does an instructor begin to develop a sense of community in an online course? Many begin with introductions or an initial request for posting of a biography. The instructor can model how the "bio" is to be posted by posting one first and asking for 1) professional experiences, 2) educational background, and 3) personal information. The "bios" will allow students to find commonalities and provide students the opportunity to get to know each other. Another technique may be to use ice breakers. Online ice breakers can include games or strategies to get students to talk about themselves, for example, "the ABC's of me" or "post eight nouns about your self". These ice breakers allow students to seek others in the class with similar interests or experiences that may facilitate good working relationships. Another strategy for facilitating community is to set up an area called cyber-chat or student lounge where students can meet and greet without loading up the main classroom with personal chatter.

ACTIVE LEARNING

In order to actively engage learners in the online learning process and to facilitate the meaning-making process that is a part of the constructivist approach through which this learning occurs, the content of the course should be embedded in everyday life (Palloff & Pratt, 1999). In other words, the more learners can relate their life experience and what they already know to the context of the online classroom, the deeper their understanding will be of what they learn. In nursing, for example, students should be provided case-based scenarios or problems to resolve based on their area of interest in nursing.

The online instructor can promote active learning through the creative use of instructional design strategies. For example, the incorporation of Web quests or problem-based learning scenarios will facilitate meaningful active learning and help students search for real life answers. A Web quest is an inquiry-oriented activity in which some or all of the information that learners interact with comes from resources on the Internet (Dodge, 1997). Web quests can be of either short or long duration and are deliberately designed to make the best use of a learner's time. Web quests should contain at least the following parts:

1. An **introduction** that sets the stage and provides some background information.
2. A **task** that is doable and interesting.
3. A set of **information sources** needed to complete the task. Many (though not necessarily all) of the resources are embedded in the Web quest document itself as anchors pointing to information on the world wide web. Information sources might include Web documents, experts available via e-mail or real-time conferencing, searchable databases on the net, and books and other documents physically available in the learner's setting. Because pointers to resources are included, the learner is not left to wander through Web space completely adrift.
4. A description of the **process** the learners should go through in accomplishing the task. The process should be broken out into clearly described steps.
5. Some **guidance** on how to organize the information acquired. This may take the form of guiding questions or directions to complete organizational frameworks such as timelines, concept maps, or cause-and-effect diagrams.
6. A **conclusion** that brings closure to the quest, reminds the learners about what they've learned, and perhaps encourages them to extend the experience into other domains.

Several examples of nursing Web quests are available on the web. For example, Nursing Organizations and Boards *http://home.dmv.com/~easycash/t-lesson-template1.htm* is a site designed for nursing students to learn about nursing organizations and roles, group work, presentations, and the Internet. This Web quest demonstrates active learning and collaborative group work while teaching students how to research and extract valuable information from the web. Another example can be found at *http://goose.ycp.edu/~dbarton/culture/*. This Web Quest teaches nursing students about culturally competent nursing care while developing research skills and group collaboration in order to complete the project.

Problem-based learning (PBL) case-based scenarios are another example of active learning strategies that can be used by instructors to promote collaboration among teams of students. PBL is an instructional method that challenges students to "learn to learn," working cooperatively in groups to seek solutions to real world problems. These problems are used to engage students' curiosity and initiate learning the subject matter. PBL prepares students to think critically and analytically, and to find and use appropriate learning resources.

With its roots in the medical profession, PBL was originally developed to assist interns to determine a diagnosis based on the given symptoms of a patient.

An example of a PBL scenario can be found on the University of Delaware Website and is titled "Who's embryo is it anyway?" *http://www.udel.edu/inst/problems/embryo/.* This case involves an ethical decision based on a mix-up at a fertility clinic. This example presents a case based on a real example and follows with four group discussion questions that require research and inquiry to answer.

Design characteristics of PBL include:

1. *Reliance on problems to drive the curriculum* — the problems do not test skills; they assist in development of the skills themselves.
2. *The problems are truly ill-structured* — there is not meant to be one solution, and as new information is gathered in a reiterative process, perception of the problem, and thus the solution, changes.
3. *Students solve the problems* — teachers are coaches and facilitators.
4. *Students are only given guidelines for how to approach problems* — there is no single formula for student approaches to the problem.
5. *Authentic, performance based assessment* — there is a seamless start and end of the instruction. (Savery & Duffy 1991).

Once students are confronted with a real world scenario they should be prompted to ask:

- What do I already know about this problem or question?
- What do I need to know to effectively address this problem or question?
- What resources can I access to determine a proposed solution or hypothesis?

When the students have clearly defined the problem, they may choose to access human or electronic information resources. They may also need to evaluate the resources by asking how current the information is, how credible and accurate it is and if there is any reason to suspect bias in the source? Since there is no assigned text in this activity, students are forced to use the Internet as the primary research tool and to critically evaluate the information they find. In the final stage, students construct a solution to the problem. Students may create a multimedia production, or a more traditional written paper focused around an essential question. This activity forces students to organize information in new ways and helps them develop new tools or strategies for solving real-world problems. In addition to developing problem-solving skills, Savery and Duffy (1991) acknowledge that students also develop skills in self-directed learning and team participation.

Cognitive apprenticeship is another strategy that involves close communication between experts and novices in an authentic context. Nurses taking clinical courses in community health, adult health or other practical areas will need to be involved in this type of learning experience. In this environment, novices progress along a path to expertise by progressively refining authentic products and processes under the mentorship of experts (Sherry, Travalin, & Billig, 2000). As with any apprenticeship, this involves observation of experts in action, coaching of novices by experts, and successive approximation to expert work as novices gain expertise. The students may be physically present in a hospital or community to develop skills while participating in the didactic part of the course online. Ongoing dialogue and conversations between and among students and instructors will help students to identify problems that they may encounter or skills that they need to develop.

SUMMARY

Interaction and communication has been identified as the core of the course where learning takes place in an online environment. It is the interaction between instructors, students and the course content that is necessary in order for the content to be applied and knowledge to be developed. Group activities and active learning techniques should be applied and are characteristic of a constructivist-learning environment. Web quests, problem-based learning and cognitive apprenticeships are examples of active learning strategies that are well-suited to the online classroom and will work well with online nursing courses.

REFERENCES

Dodge, B. (1997). *The web quest page.* Retrieved January 29, 2003, from http://Web quest.sdsu.edu/

Gilbert, S. D. (2001). *How to be a successful online student.* NewYork, NY: McGraw Hill professional, New York.

Palloff, R. & Pratt, K. (1999). *Building learning communities in cyberspace: Effective strategies for the online classroom.* San-Francisco: Jossey-Bass.

Picciano, A. (2001). *Distance learning: Making connections across virtual space and time.* Old Tappen, NJ: Prentice Hall

Sherry, L., Traralin, F., & Billig, S. (2000). Good online conversation: Building on research to inform practice. *Journal of Interactive Learning Research,* 11(1), 85–127.

Savery, J., & Duffy, T. (1991). *Problem Based Learning.* In B. Wilson, Constructivist learning environments: Case studies in instructional design (pp. 135–146). Englewood Cliffs, NJ:Educational Technology Publications.

9

Assessment and Evaluation of Online Learning

"Learning involves changing to a new state—it is a state that persists, what can be learned? New thinking strategies, new motor skills, and new attitudes are learned in complex patterns that can promote a new performance" (Redman, 2001, p.21). Assessing the learner is the gathering of data to identify needs, ability, progress, and resources. Assessment is student oriented and is used to place, promote, graduate, and/or retain students.

Evaluation is a judgment made by comparing a behavior to a standard. Evaluation is the measurement of a behavior and the comparison of that behavior to a predetermined expectation.

ASSESSMENT, EVALUATION, AND PEDAGOGY

Pedagogical theory forms the framework for the design of a learning experience. Learning objectives, learning strategies, and evaluation activities flow from the pedagogical theory. For example, if the theory used to design a learning experience were behavioral theory, you expect to see learning objectives that focus on the targeted behavior and strategies that include rewards and consequences. The objectives and strategies drive the evaluation activities. If the learning objective is to state five signs and symptoms of congestive heart failure, the evaluation should measure that the learner can state the signs and symptoms. To determine if the student has achieved this objective, the student may be asked to name five signs and symptoms of congestive heart failure or may be asked to answer a multiple-choice question.

TRADITIONAL ASSESSMENT AND EVALUATION

A traditional evaluation design measures the attainment of learning objectives through exams, papers, and projects that the student submits to the instructor. The instructor uses criteria to grade the student's assignments and to categorize them into a grade of "A," "B," etc. The student demonstrates learning as stipulated in the objectives, and based on the degree of attainment of those objectives, a grade is assigned. This is called norm-referenced assessment because we make judgments about learning and a bell-shaped curve is an expected outcome. This means that some students get D's and F's and others get A's and the mean is about a B or C. The students are responsible for their learning and their grade. Another type of assessment is criterion-referenced which is based on learning for the purpose of meeting a standard. In this type of assessment, the instructor is responsible for helping all learners meet the standard. An example of a standard is validation, such as CPR validation.

In addition to the students, traditional evaluation includes gathering data about the course from an end-of-course survey that is completed by students. Data is compiled and sometime after the end of the course, the data is given to the faculty to review. Data may be used to make changes in the course delivery before the next time it is offered.

Traditional assessments may also include measuring the student's progress through a course or on the way to completing the course. Usually assessment techniques are process oriented and might take the form of a quiz. The purpose of assessment is to check the progress of students to identify those who may be struggling through the course.

The Committee on the Foundations of Assessment (Pellegrino, Chudowsky, Glasser, 2001) expressed their concern that assessment practices in current use only partially meet the goals of informing and improving education. The Committee concluded that assessment practices have changed over time but have not kept up with the changes in learning models and theories. They report that the basic knowledge base of assessment is available but needs to be put into practice and expanded. The purpose of this chapter is to expand the base knowledge of assessment and evaluation and expand this knowledge into online learning environments.

CONSTRUCTIVISM AND ONLINE LEARNING

When constructivism is the guiding theory in learning, students construct new knowledge by actively engaging in learning strategies. Students reflect on the learned content and their reflections bring meaning to a larger social context or solve real-world problems. Learning is process oriented and when basic knowledge is used to construct new knowledge, the basic knowledge is reinforced. Traditional evaluation designs that predominantly focus on measuring the student's learning of objectives will not provide a comprehensive picture of the student's learning. Focusing on the student's learning process while they are constructing new knowledge is important. While learners are constructing new knowledge, they need feedback. Feedback means that learners need comments from teachers that will motivate them to continue constructing knowledge or to continue moving in a constructive direction.

A traditional evaluation design does not accommodate the use of technology as a learning tool. Let's say that a student registers for a fully Web-based course and shows up at the faculty's office the second week of the semester asking where the class will be held. Somehow, the student already has missed information and thus progress is hampered. By the second week of the semester, the student should have the computer skills needed to negotiate the online course; should have the needed resources (i.e. course entry information such as user name and password), and should know how to navigate through the course. If the student does not have these basic skills, the student will have to spend time learning navigational skills instead of course material. To get the student directly into the learning material, precourse student assessments should be planned into the design of the learning experiences. These assessments should provide data about the student's readiness to take a course online. Data gathered about the student's readiness should be summarized and a prescriptive plan should be developed that will guide the learner to resources needed to be successful online. The prescriptive plan is written and individualized for each student. The plan includes activities and outcomes that focus on the skills that will ensure success online. Some examples include: knowing how to download files, navigating the Web, receiving and sending e-mail, sending attachments, and basic typing skills.

When developing learning material online, the learning material should be peer reviewed before it is released to learners. A peer review is a process in which a designated reviewer uses established criteria to review a course.

Information gathered from the review is shared with the course developers so corrections can be made before students log on to the course. A peer review is crucial for newly developed courses because there may be links that do not work, there may be spelling and grammar errors, or there may be exam dates in the syllabus that are not the same as the dates on a calendar. The purpose of a peer review is to enhance the quality of learning.

The reviewer has a "fresh set of eyes" that can detect glaring errors so they can be corrected before the learners arrive. It is recommended that peers review or follow a course while it is offered to students. Faculty should be recognized for their contributions and successes when they teach online. Faculty who teach online should ask content and technology experts to "sit-in" on their courses as guests to provide feedback for the faculty. The feedback can be used for tenure and promotion, to promote recognition of scholarship of teaching and learning online, and to provide visibility for online courses especially to faculty who do not teach online.

Technology has influences on the course before it is offered, while it is being offered, and at the end of the course. Online learners need an orientation to the technology and learning platform before the course starts. Evaluating the effectiveness of the orientation is important for revising and refining. During the course, servers can crash and hard drives can go down. During one semester students were assigned to gather secondary data about a community. Data about the behavioral indicators of a community, such as smoking, obesity, prenatal care, etc., which were located on a server that was managed by the state health department. About a week before starting content on the community assessment module, the information was pulled off line by the state health department. The faculty checked the links to this Web site before the course started, so the faculty did not know the link was not working when the students were working on the assignment. But the students knew and the e-mails from students to faculty increased. So evaluating the online course while it is live is essential. Early in the course, the faculty can ask students to e-mail them with anything that looks like a course issue as soon as it becomes apparent. Give students permission to ask "dumb" questions like "Should the syllabus icon go to the syllabus?" Faculty needs information to quickly correct the "glitches". Aside from technical issues, there could be learner issues. Conflicts between students may develop or there could be hurt feelings because someone typed something that someone else read as negative. A quick response to technical and student issues while the course is running prevents further (and usually more chaotic) repercussions. At the end, the course needs to be evaluated by faculty, learners, and instructional designers using tools that focus on gathering data that is particular to online courses.

SUMMARY OF TRADITIONAL VS. ONLINE ASSESSMENT AND EVALUATION

In summary, evaluation of online learning differs from that of traditional classroom learning. Assessing the learner is an essential component in online learning. Learner skills and ability need to be assessed, learner's response to orientation needs to be assessed, learners need feedback during the course while they are constructing new knowledge, and learners need grades assigned at the end of the course. Therefore, traditional assessment and evaluation models need to be revised to accommodate learning online.

FOUNDATIONAL KNOWLEDGE ON ASSESSMENT AND EVALUATION

The Committee on the Foundations of Assessment (Pellegrino, Ludowsky, Glasser 2001) depicts the foundational knowledge on assessment and evaluation as a triangle with three key elements: cognition, observation, and interpretation. These three elements are connected to and dependent on each other. Cognition is defined as the aspects of achievement that will be assessed. Observation is the collecting of evidence about the student's achievement. Interpretation is the methods used to analyze the collected evidence.

Smith and Ragan (1999) use the term "evaluation". They offer two purposes of evaluation: to assess individual students' performances and to provide information to revise course material. Smith and Ragan call evaluation a way of "getting there": Did the student "get there" and how well did the instruction get the student there. They suggest that assessments be based on the learning objectives and such assessments are called criterion-referenced assessment items. Their purpose is to assess competence or to identify gaps in learning. But they do not compare or rank learners. That is the purpose of norm-referenced tests. Smith and Ragan write that assessments are either criterion or norm referenced, thus alluding to two types of assessment: to identify gaps and to compare students learning.

They describe three types of assessments: entry skills assessments, preassessments, and postassessments. The entry skills assessment focuses on skills needed to be successful in the online course; preassessments focus on ascertaining what the students already know, and postassessments focus on attainment of learning objectives. They outline characteristics of good assessment instruments as: validity, reliability, and practicality. A valid assessment answers the question: Does it measure what it claims it will measure? A reliable instrument is one that yields consistent outcomes over time. A practical assessment is cost effective. Smith and Ragan suggest two formats of assessment: performance assessment and paper-and-pencil tests.

Smith and Ragan further describe evaluation as a means of providing information to revise course material and offers two types of evaluation: formative and summative. Formative evaluations provide information for the purpose of revising the instruction, and summative evaluations provide data about the continued use of the instruction.

NEW MODEL FOR ASSESSING AND EVALUATING ONLINE LEARNING

The authors of this book developed a model that incorporates the foundations of assessment and evaluation, guided constructivism and online learning. The following questions were asked: Did the teaching methods and strategies used in this learning experience effectively impart information? Did the recipients learn the information? These questions are answered when assessing student learning and evaluating the course.

Assessment and evaluation are activities that are planned when the course is designed. The activities should be appropriate and congruous measures of the goals and objectives of the course. The activities provide data that can be used to make judgments about student learning and course effectiveness. Data can be gathered about the feasibility of student success online, the progress of the student through the course, student achievement of the course objectives at the end of the course, the effectiveness of the course design, the effectiveness of the course while it is taught and the outcomes of the course. Student learning and course functioning are two aspects that need to be addressed separately. A model is suggested that will focus on student learning and course evaluations separately.

Assessment focuses on the student and evaluation focuses on the course. Assessment and evaluation are built into the course design and are visible throughout the course from the precourse, through the course; at the end of the course.

Assessment is defined as the identification of student needs and progress throughout the learning experience. The purpose of precourse assessments is to identify the needs of the student so they can be remediated before the course begins. During the course, the focus is on the student's progress. The faculty monitors the student throughout the course and gives feedback about the process of constructing new knowledge. Assessing the learner at the end of the course is determined by graded activities. Grading criteria should be clearly specified in the syllabus.

Evaluation focuses on the course itself. Precourse evaluation includes peer review of the course and an evaluation of the orientation program that is given to students before they enter the course. Forma-

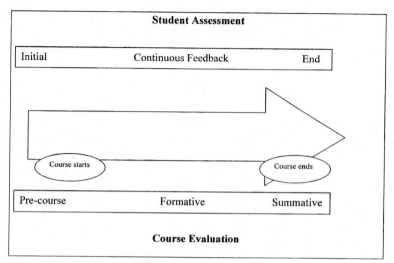

FIGURE 9.1 The model for assessing and evaluating learning online.

tive evaluation is directed at how the course is operating and summative evaluation is evaluation of the course after it is completed.

A new model called The Model for Assessing and Evaluating Learning Online as seen in Figure 9.1 was developed based on Smith and Ragan (1999) and the Assessment Triangle. The aspects of achievement (cognition) are divided into three phases for student assessment and three phases of course evaluation.

During each phase evidence is gathered and analyzed. At each phase decisions are made based on the analyzed evidence. For example, at the end of the initial phase of student assessment, a prescriptive plan is developed which outlines knowledge and competencies that the student needs to master to continue in the course. During the continuous assessment, students are given feedback and motivation to help them determine their progress. The end student assessment is the measure of individual achievement. Evidence is gathered about the student's ability to meet objectives and a decision to pass or fail is determined.

STUDENT INITIAL ASSESSMENT

Various types of initial student assessment techniques have been identified. These techniques can be used to determine a range of student skills from comfort with technology to preferred learning styles. The following list* includes some suggestions for faculty to use when conducting an initial student assessment prior to participating in an online course:

- Initial letter of assessment about themselves as a learner
- Placement exams
- Students develop personal Web pages
- Electronic meeting
- Computer skills exercise
- Pretests
- Scavenger hunt to assess navigation skills, (develop a scavenger hunt list and posting of announcements; ask students to 'find' the items and e-mail the answers to the instructor)
- Learning style surveys
- Readiness surveys

CONTINUOUS FEEDBACK

Continuous student feedback can be conducted at any time during the course. The purpose of continuous feedback is to determine if the student is learning from the course material presented. It is important for the faculty to know if the lectures and content of the course have been presented in a clear and logical format. Obtaining this information prior to the end of the course enables the instructor to make changes. Some of these techniques* include:

- Journaling, writing marathons, diaries: techniques to assess attitude and satisfaction (affective objectives); written logs about experiences and reflections
- Concept map: connective key concepts
- Mid-semester assessment
- Estimating student time ranges for each assignment plus interaction
- Feedback
- Three-minute "things I don't understand about_____"
- Weekly new idea
- Debate

- Students answer the question: What was the fuzziest point?
- Reaction paper
- Worksheets
- Nongraded quizzes
- Simulations
- Crossword puzzles
- Attendance
- Peer questions to other students
- Participation in discussion board
- Homework assignments
- Questioning
- Case studies: detailed accounts of a client, family, group (pregnant teens) or community.

END STUDENT ASSESSMENT

At the end of a course, students are assessed in terms of meeting the course learning objectives. Multiple methods can be used and the following list identifies some methods:

- Quizzes
- Compositions, essays, and papers
- Projects (individual or group); project summaries
- Web-page presentations
- Analysis of newspaper article
- Examinations: exams can be multiple choice and/or essay. Exams can be timed and proctored to ensure that students submit their own work. Students can take exams in schools of nursing, at outreach sites, at community colleges with faculty proctors, at local libraries, or at home with approved proctors. Exams can be proctored at testing centers such as the Sylvan Learning Centers. Proctoring by video may also be an option.
- Portfolios: called e-folios, which are collections of student work in the course stored in a digital medium such as a CD. The work may include reflective essays, patient care plans, pamphlets developed for a health fair, pictures of a health-project at an immunization fair, or an audiotape of a song to prevent teen pregnancy.

- Student presentations
- Peer evaluation
- Final interviews

Rubrics are sets of standards that can be used to assign grades and give students feedback about their performance. Rubrics can use descriptions or commentaries on achievement, such as excellent, good, fair, poor, they can be based on competencies and they can address multidimensional skills such as a group project (Huba & Freed, 2000). Anderson, Bauer, and Speck (2002) provide examples of rubrics that can be used to assess student work in chat rooms, bulletin boards, on written or group projects and in field experiences. An abbreviated rubric for assessing chat room participation (Anderson, Bauer & Speck, 2002, p. 33) is:

9–10 points for logging into chatroom on time and fully participating in discussions
7–8 points for logging in with variable participation in discussions
5–6 points for logging in late and participating infrequently in discussions
1–4 points for missing chats and rarely participating in discussions

PRECOURSE EVALUATION

Precourse evaluation helps faculty to determine if the course is ready for launching. An external, objective reviewer should ideally review the course for content and for instructional design. The peer reviewer should then continue to observe the course for interaction approximately two weeks into the course and again at midterm. The reviewer should provide constructive feedback to the instructor, which can be used to make changes in the course. Pre-evaluation activities can include:

- Peer review of content
- Peer review of design
- Ongoing peer review

- Course review by students
- Evaluation of orientation to online learning

Fellows in the Web Initiative in Teaching Project (WIT, a University System of Maryland faculty initiative, 1998—2002) developed a Peer Review Process for new online courses. Margaret Chambers (*http://www.mindlinked.com*), Director of the Institute of Distance Education at the University of Maryland University College and the Web Initiative in Teaching Project, wrote the following letter to external peer reviewers to describe the peer review process. The peer review criteria can be found in Appendix A.

The WIT peer review process was developed in response to concerns of tenure track faculty who wish to receive recognition for the scholarship of teaching that is needed to create and teach a successful Web-based course. Throughout the developmental process we have engaged in peer feedback using an evolving set of criteria or profiling characteristics (see the bottom of this message). This external review of the teaching pilot is intended to ascertain the overall quality of the Web course to facilitate active learning and interaction. Each WIT external peer review committee will consist of two discipline specialists and will be coordinated by a WIT Fellow from another institution who successfully authored and taught a Web-based course the previous year.

Each peer review committee will receive a set of review questions based on the profiling categories and will be asked to complete two questionnaires, one in early October and the other at the end of the semester. By the end of January, the team will be asked to submit a brief narrative report(s) based upon the review questions/categories. Unlike a face-to-face classroom, the Web-enabled virtual classroom is open for your observations throughout the semester at your convenience. We are asking that you make an initial visit to the course Web site at the beginning of the semester, acquainting yourself with the syllabus and structure of the course, visiting the interactive conferencing, and testing the ease and logic of navigation around the Web course site. We will send you an electronic questionnaire the third week in September to gather your initial observations.

Asynchronous discussions unfold over time. We would like to have you visit the course for an entire week at least once in order to observe the pacing and style of learning interactions. An alternative might be to select and follow a module from the beginning to the end. Some of you may "shadow" the course on a weekly basis throughout the semester. The key is that you observe sufficiently to get an accurate reading of the quality of the interaction between the instructor and the students, and among the students.

Your final questionnaire will be sent around Thanksgiving and will be due by December 15. A short narrative report from the team as a whole or from individuals will be due by January 15.

You will receive instructions on how to access your Web course immediately from the course instructor. We hope you will find this experience broadens your knowledge and appreciation of teaching on the Web. On behalf of all the WIT Project participants, I want to thank you for your willingness to participate in this undertaking.
Margaret Chambers
Director

FORMATIVE EVALUATION

Formative evaluation throughout the course allows the faculty to determine if course delivery, structure,- or instructional design needs revising. For example, students may ask for a discussion forum to list technology issues and ask for peer help. By providing students with the opportunity to ask questions during the course, issues can be resolved quickly and students can focus on their learning. Some suggestions for formative evaluation are:

- "Pulse Check": ask students on a regular basis, maybe every four weeks or three times during the semester, to post or email their "pulse" — where they are and how they are doing in the course and what improvements or changes they think should be made
- Discussion summaries every other week about course content and issues
- Mid-semester survey
- Verbal feedback to specific questions

SUMMATIVE EVALUATION

The institution often requires summative evaluation. This evaluation provides feedback to the faculty to revise the course and to evaluate the faculty. Examples include:

- Student evaluation of course
- Student evaluation of faculty
- Faculty evaluation of course

The Web Initiative in Teaching Fellows in the WIT Project developed a pool of questions based on the categories of an effective online course. Questions were developed for three audiences: the reviewer, the instructor, and the student. You can use this pool by first choosing your audience. If you are developing a survey for students as an end-of-course survey, look in the student column of the Pool of Potential Items in Appendix B. Read the items and choose the ones that are reflective and pertinent to your student population. Including items from each category will enhance the validity of the survey.

California State University, Chico's (2002) Committee for Evaluation of Exemplary Online Courses has developed a rubric to identify a quality online course. The criteria include: online organization and design, instructional design and delivery, assessment and evaluation of student learning, appropriate and effective use of technology, and learner support and resources. Baseline, effective, and exemplary quality are delineated.

SUMMARY

A model has been developed that can be used to assess student learning and evaluate the learning environment. It incorporates the foundations of assessment and evaluation, guided constructivism, and online learning. Students should be assessed before the course starts to determine needs and learning style, during the course to determine progress, and at the end of the course as a final assessment of attaining goals. The course is peer evaluated before it is opened to students. Frequent evaluation of the course while it is being offered helps to identify problems and issues that can be remedied. Evaluating the course at the end provides data to revise the course and data that can be used in developing new courses.

*Developed in collaboration with participants at the Lilly Conference, Towson University, Baltimore, Maryland, April 2002.

REFERENCES

Anderson, R.S., Bauer, J.F., & Speck, B.W. (2002). *Assessment strategies for the on-line class: From theory to practice.* San Francisco: Jossey-Bass.

California State University, Chico. *Rubric for online instruction.* Retrieved February 3, 2003, from http://*www.csuchico.edu/tlp/webct/rubric/rubric_final.pdf.*

Huba, M.E. & Freed, J.E. (2000). *Learner-centered assessment on college campuses: Shifting the focus from teaching to learning.* Boston, MA: Allen and Bacon Publishers.

Pellegrino J.W., Chudowsky, N., Glasser, R. (2001) Knowing What Students Know: The science and design of educational assessment. Retrieved October 1, 2003 from *http://www.nap.edu/open book/0309072727/html/r6.html.*

Redman, B.K. (2001) The Practice of Patient Education. St. Louis, MO: Mosby, Inc.

Smith. P. & Ragan, T. (1999). *Instructional Design* (2nd ed.). New York: John Wiley & Sons, Inc.

Table 9.1 Criteria for Peer Review of Online Courses*

The Web Course Profiling Categories

PART ONE: Review of the Course Design and Implementation

1. Course rationale and syllabus
2. Goals and objectives
3. Instructional design for Web environments
4. Theoretical basis for learning and teaching (pedagogical foundations)
5. Content and metacontent
6. Learning and teaching strategies and activities
7. Interactivity and community building (with faculty, students, and content)
8. Use of mediated resources, electronic libraries, and the Web
9. Orientation, induction into online learning, metalearning (learning how to learn online)
10. Responsiveness to learner needs (learning-centric, learner sensitive)
11. Diversity, multiple cultural perspectives, accommodation for geographic distance
12. Assessment and evaluation
13. Accessibility, robustness, and technical support (Infrastructure and ease of use for instructor and students)
14. Interface design and navigation
15. Intellectual property: copyright, attribution, rights for use
16. Internal organization and consistency ** (OVERRIDING CRITERIA)

PART TWO: Review of Pilot Delivery & Teaching Effectiveness

17. Instructor's role and teaching effectiveness
18. Students' levels of engagement, motivation, achievement, and satisfaction

---

*Developed by the Web Initiative in Teaching Fellows, University System of Maryland

TABLE 9.2 Web initiative in Teaching—Pool of Potential Items to Evaluate Online Courses: Potential Items Appropriate to the Reviewer, the Teacher, and the Student of Online Courses

Category	Reviewer	Teacher	Student
Course rationale	The purpose of the course is stated The purpose is clear The purpose is appropriate The purpose described how this course fit into the curriculum	Same	Same
Learning and teaching theories	The use of a specific theory is evident The theory is used consistently in course development The theory is used consistently in course implementation	The underlying theory used to develop the course was evident The theory used to develop the course was appropriate for the content and the student The theory was easy to implement	New approaches to learning were used in this course
Goals and objectives	Explicit learning goals were included in this course Learning goals were clearly specified Learning goals were skill oriented Learning goals were knowledge oriented Learning goals were process oriented Learning goals were available throughout the course The learning goals could be easily found in the course material	Same	Same

TABLE 9.2 (*Continued*)

Category	Reviewer	Teacher	Student
Learning strategies	The instructional activities were clearly related to the learning goals	The instructional activities were clearly related to the learning goals	Same as Reviewer
	The required readings contributed to skill or knowledge acquisition	The material was sequenced to facilitate learning	
	The required asynchronous discussion or conferencing contributed to knowledge acquisition	The students were able to choose the sequencing of the material	
	The required video materials contributed to skill/knowledge/experience acquisition	Differences in learning styles were accounted for in designing the course activities	
	The required chat or synchronous discussion contributed to knowledge acquisition	The course design stresses the importance of goals and objectives that exist apart from the learner	
	The required guest lectures contributed to skill/knowledge/experience acquisition	The course design emphasizes the primacy of the learners intentions and experience	
	The material was sequenced to facilitate learning	The instructor's role is different from that in a face-to-face course	
	The students were able to choose the sequencing of the material		
	Differences in learning styles were accounted for in designing the course activities		
	The course design stresses the importance of goals and objectives that exist apart from the learner		
	The instructor's role is different from that in a face-to-face course		

TABLE 9.2 (*Continued*)

Category	Reviewer	Teacher	Student
Instructional design	The course delivery system is flexible enough to meet this course's needs The course material is appropriately designed to provide opportunities for timely feedback by learners The course design allows for timely feedback by learners on course delivery, including technology and support services The course design allows for timely feedback by learners on instructor accessibility When appropriate, the course design allows for anonymous feedback	Same as Reviewer	The course delivery system is flexible enough to meet this course's needs
Content	The course material is appropriately designed to provide opportunities for timely feedback by learners The course design allows for timely feedback by learners on course delivery, including technology and support services The course design allows for timely feedback by learners on instructor accessibility	Content was appropriate for meeting learning objectives Content is scholarly Content is integrated into new teaching methods There is evidence of original conception of content and strategy New novel teaching materials were generated	The course material is appropriately designed to provide opportunities for timely feedback by learners The course design allows for timely feedback by learners on course delivery,

TABLE 9.2 (*Continued*)

Category	Reviewer	Teacher	Student
Content (*cont.*)	When appropriate, the course design allows for anonymous feedback Content is scholarly Content is integrated into new teaching methods There is evidence of original conception of content and strategy New novel teaching materials were generated New novel content was generated	New novel content was generated	including technology and support services The course design allows for timely feedback by learners on instructor accessibility When appropriate, the course design allows for anonymous feedback
Interactivity	Synchronous student to student interaction is an important part of this course Asynchronous student to student interaction is an important part of this course Too much time is spent on student interaction in this course Student to student interaction is clearly linked to the learning goals Student to student interaction is flexible enough to accommodate different learning styles in this course	Synchronous student to student interaction is an important part of this course Asynchronous student to student interaction is an important part of this course Too much time is spent on student interaction in this course Student to student interaction is clearly linked to the learning goals Student to student interaction is flexible enough to accommodate different learning styles in this course	Synchronous student to student interaction is an important part of this course Asynchronous student to student interaction is an important part of this course Student to student interaction is clearly linked to the learning goals Student to student interaction is flexible enough to accommodate different learning styles in this course

TABLE 9.2 (*Continued*)

Category	Reviewer	Teacher	Student
Interactivity (*cont.*)	The instructor helped to facilitate student to student interaction	I played an important part in student to student interaction	course
	The instructor's moderation of asynchronous interaction was effective	My moderation of asynchronous interaction was effective	The instructor helped to facilitate student to student interaction
	The instructor's moderation of asynchronous interaction increased understanding of the content	My moderation of asynchronous interaction increased understanding of the content	The instructor's moderation of asynchronous interaction was effective
	A policy on the instructor's response time to student e-mail was in place	I consistently met my policy on response time to student e-mails	The instructor's moderation of asynchronous interaction increased understanding of the content
	A policy on the instructor's response time to student conferencing questions was in place	I consistently met my policy on response time to student conferencing questions	A policy on the instructor's response time to student e-mail was in place
	The instructor's response to student questions were consistently helpful	My responses to student questions were helpful	A policy on the instructor's response time to student conferencing questions was in place
	The policy on the response time to student e-mail was appropriate	Interacting with the students was burdensome	The instructor followed the policy on response time to student emails
	The policy on the response time to student conferencing questions was appropriate	Interacting with the students took more time than I expected	The instructor followed the policy on response time to student conferencing questions
	The interaction in this class appeared to be excessive	The interaction in this class appeared to be excessive	The instructor's response to student questions
	The student's ability to use the technology affected interaction	The student's ability to use the technology affected interaction between students	
	Class assignments encouraged interaction between students	Class assignments encouraged interaction between students	

TABLE 9.2 (Continued)

Category	Reviewer	Teacher	Student
Interactivity (*cont.*)			were consistently helpful Interacting with the instructor was burdensome Interacting with the instructor and other students took more time than I expected My ability to use technology affected my interaction with the instructor and other students Class assignments encouraged interaction between students
Use of technology resources	The use of instructional technologies was consistent with the objectives of the course The use of instructional technologies was consistent with the required assignments The assessments were appropriate to instructional technologies used The required plug-ins for the course were clearly identified and downloaded	Same as Reviewer	The required plug-ins for the course were clearly identified and downloaded I was adequately prepared for the instructional technology used in this course I had access to technical support for the instructional technology used in this course

TABLE 9.2 *(Continued)*

Category	Reviewer	Teacher	Student
	The combined instructional technologies in this course were capable of creating a learning community		My level of technical expertise with computers and the internet at the start of the course was sufficient
	The required tasks in this course could not have been accomplished without incorporating instructional technologies		My computer required a hardware upgrade for me to take this course online
	The combined instructional technologies improved the instructional quality of the course		
	The instructional technologies of this course were effectively utilized		
	The instructional technology facilitated faculty student rapport		
Accessibility, robustness, and technical support		Support services were readily available to help me with course development	
		Technical support services were easily accessible	
		Technical support services were always available	
		Technical support services were adequate	

TABLE 9.2 (*Continued*)

Category	Reviewer	Teacher	Student
Accessibility, robustness, and technical support (*cont.*)		Technical support services were effective	My computer required a software upgrade for me to take this course online
		I know or can easily find whom to call if I have a technical problem	The required video materials contributed to skill/knowledge/experience acquisition
		The response time by technical services was short	A tutorial was available on navigating the course
		There is a comprehensive system of technical support services	The upgrade of the hardware was difficult or time consuming
		Support services are offered 7 days a week, 24 hours a day	Technical support services were easily accessible
			Technical support services were adequate
			Technical support services were effective
			I know or can easily find whom to call if I have a technical problem
			The response time by technical services was short
Navigation	It was easy to get around the course	It was easy to get around the course	It was easy to get around the course

TABLE 9.2 (*Continued*)

Category	Reviewer	Teacher	Student
Assessment and evaluation	Students had an opportunity to assess the peer interaction in this course	Students had an opportunity to assess the peer interaction in this course	Students had an opportunity to assess the peer interaction in this course
	The student to student interaction in this course created a sense of community	The student to student interaction in this course created a sense of community	The student to student interaction in this course created a sense of community
	The student to student interaction in this course created a greater sense of community than in a traditional face to face course	The student to student interaction in this course created a greater sense of community than in a traditional face to face course	The student to student interaction in this course created a greater sense of community than in a traditional face to face course
	Assessment instruments are consistent with the learning goals	Assessment instruments are consistent with the learning goals	Assessment instruments are consistent with the learning goals
	Assessment instruments evaluate the skills the learner is expected to master	Assessment instruments evaluate the skills the learner is expected to master	Assessment instruments evaluate the skills the learner is expected to master
	Assessment instruments evaluate the concepts the learner is expected to master	Assessment instruments evaluate the concepts the learner is expected to master	Assessment instruments evaluate the concepts the learner is expected to master
	Assessment instruments evaluate the knowledge the learner is expected to master	Assessment instruments evaluate the knowledge the learner is expected to master	Assessment instruments evaluate the knowledge the learner is expected to master
	Assessment instruments require the same skills as learning activities	Assessment instruments require the same skills as learning activities	
	Assessment instruments require the same concepts as learning activities	Assessment instruments require the same concepts as learning activities	
	Assessment instruments require the same knowledge as learning activities		

TABLE 9.2 (Continued)

Category	Reviewer	Teacher	Student
Assessment and evaluation (cont.)	Assessment and measurement strategies accommodate individual special need of learners Assessment and measurement strategies are sufficiently flexible to accommodate the learner's unique situation Assessment criteria for web-based assignments were explicit An externally administered, criteria referenced assessment instrument was used	Assessment instruments require the same knowledge as learning activities Assessment and measurement strategies accommodate individual special need of learners Assessment and measurement strategies are sufficiently flexible to accommodate the learner's unique situation Assessment criteria for web-based assignments were explicit An externally administered, criteria referenced assessment instrument was used	Assessment instruments require the same skills as learning activities Assessment instruments require the same concepts as learning activities Assessment instruments require the same knowledge as learning activities Assessment instruments were integral to your experience Assessment instruments enabled you to evaluate your own progress Assessment instruments enabled you to identify areas for review Assessment and measurement strategies accommodated my individual special needs

TABLE 9.2 (*Continued*)

Category	Reviewer	Teacher	Student
Assessment and evaluation (*cont.*)			Assessment and measurement strategies were sufficiently flexible to accommodate my unique situation The instructor was explicit on his/her assessment criteria for web-based assignments An externally administered, criteria referenced assessment instrument was used
Instructor's Effectiveness			The instructor was actively involved in the course The instructor helped me learn The instructor guided my learning

Developed by the University System of Maryland WIT Fellows, 1999.

Index

A

AACN
Aceware® Systems, 35
Active dialogue, 128
Active learning, 4, 20, 22, 88, 131–132
Active participation, 128
Advising students
  Asynchronous and synchronous advising, 36
  Advisors web page guidelines, 38
  National Academic Advising Association (NACADA), 29, 37–38
Agenda
  Course, 105
  Weekly, 105
American Association of Colleges of Nursing (AACN)
  And technology supported education, 28
  Whitepaper, 9
Americans with Disabilities Act (ADA)
  Bobby TM approved, 110–111
Angel software, 40
Announcements (see course announcements)
Animation, use of, 127
Assignments
  Group, 104–106
  Individual, 104–106
  Weekly, 104–106

Assessment
  Criterion referenced, 138, 142
  Model, 144
  Norm referenced, 138, 142
  Traditional, 138
Assess the learner (or target population), 82
Association of College and Research Libraries (ACRL) guidelines, 35
Asynchronous communication (see also asynchronous interaction), 2
Asynchronous interaction, 1–4, 15–16, 21, 51, 92, 126
Asynchronous Learning Networks, 2, 94
Automation, 5
Audio technology (see also voice technology), 27

B

Banner® software, 35
Blackboard® courseware, 40, 49, 52, 56, 94
  Biosketch, 131
Blended learning, 66–67

C

California Virtual University, 2
Case studies, 21, 67, 88, 132
Chat room, 51, 129, 49
Clinical courses, 63, 74–76
Commercialism of higher education, 6
Communication (see synchronous, asynchronous and interaction)

Community building, 130
  Also see learning teams
  Collaboration, 15, 30, 99–100,
    130, 131
Conflicts, student, 141
Cognitive apprenticeship, 134
Constructivism (see Theories in
  education),
Consumer health informatics, 6–7
Content, organizing, 85
Continuing education, 8
Conversation, online, 126
Copyright Law, 28, 41, 42, 44–45
Course
  Agenda, 105
  Americans with Disabilities Act
    considerations, 110–111
  Announcements, 103
  Assignments, 104
  Directions, 104
  Documents, 104
  Management, 51
  Pace, 106
  Planning, 51
  Requirements, 102
Course content, chunking, 86
Course information, general, 102–
  103

D

Data technology, 48
Design models
  Checklist, 88
  Linear Mode with star nodes
    attached, 88
  Spread, 87
Design support, 51
Discussion area (also see
  asynchronous), 49, 126–128
Discussion questions, 83, 92, 99
Distance education technologies
  (see print technology, voice
  technology and data
  technology)
Diversity consideration, 109

E

Education Review Technology Source,
  2
Educause, 2
E-learn, 56
Electronic mail (E-mail), 4, 49, 51,
  126
Evaluation of course
  Criteria, 153–163
  Formative evaluation, 149
  Model, 144
  Precourse evaluation, 147–148
  Summative evaluation, 149–150
  Traditional, 138
Excelsior College, 47
Expansive questioning, 99–100
Expectations, students (see student
  learning)

F

Faculty role, 97
  As community builder, 130
  As facilitator (see also interaction,
    faculty to student), 16
  Characteristics, 24
  Competencies, 54
  Responsibilities of, 97–98
  Tenure and promotion, 140
Faculty support
  Training, Indiana Higher Education
    Telecommunications System
    (IHETS) recommendations, 40,
    55
  Training for student advising,
    NACADA standards, 42
  Technical, and collaboration
    with information technology, 40,
    55
  Workload definition, 15, 40, 41
Fair Use Law, 44–45
Feedback, 4, 73, 104, 106–108, 139,
  143–144, 155–156
Fund for the Improvement of Post
  Secondary Education (FISPS), 6

G

Glossary, 51
Grading, 49, 104–105
Graphics, use of, 127
Groups, 128
Guided constructivism, 22, 25, 80,
    81–82, 143

H

Hybrid (also see blended learning), 1,
    60, 65–66

I

Ice breaker, 8, 88, 99, 131
Illinois Online network (ION), 16,
    98, 113, 115
Institutional considerations
    Commitment, 30
    Financial, 28–29
    Library services, 35–36
    Mission statement, 27, 29
    NACADA standards, 29–30
    Policies, 30
    Recruiting students, 28, 29
    Strategic plan, 27, 29
    Technological, 30
Infrastructure, definition of, 27
Informatics competencies, 54
Instructional design, definition of, 79
Instructional enhancement initiative, 6
Intellectual property, 28, 41
Interaction, 125
    Faculty to student, 97–99
    Student to student, 127
    Groups, 127
Internet etiquette (see netiquette)
Internet Equity & Education Act of
    2001, 34
Iowa Communication Network
    (ICN), 31

L

Laboratory courses, 63, 73
Learning anytime anywhere
    partnerships (LAAP), 6

Learning activities, 88–89
Learning styles, types of, 83
    Auditory/verbal learner, 84
    Assessment of and the ION, 83
    Tactile/kinesthetic, 84
    Visual/non-verbal, 5, 84
    Visual/verbal, 84
Learning teams (see also interaction
    between groups), 128–129
Lotus Learning Space®, 49, 52, 55,
    56

M

Managing an online course
    Academic honesty, 121
    Attendance, 120
    Grading, 120–122
    Group work, 120–127
    Late assignments, 120
    Participation, 120
    Schedule, 123
Mental models, 19, 68, 71, 85, 86,
    94
Multimedia, 15, 89, 127, 134

N

National Academic Advising
    Association (NACADA)
    standards, 29, 37
Navigation and page layout, 90–91,
    126
Netiquette, 108–109
Newsgroups, 20
No significant difference
    phenomenon, 3

O

Objectives, writing, 84
Online delivery systems, types of
    (also see BlackBoard, WEB CT,
    Lotus Learning Space), 50–52
Online grading, 51
Online help (see technical assistance),
Online instruction, 1
Online learning, 13–16

Online self-helpers, 7
Online testing requirements, 51
Outlook Express®, 56

P

Page layout guidelines, 90–91
Participation guidelines, 129
Peer review, 140–148, 152
Pennsylvania State University, 2, 27, 84
People soft®, 35
Portfolio, 146
Power Point®, 54, 127
Prescriptive plan, 140, 144
Principles and practice for the design and development of distance education, 84–85
Principles for good practice, 5–Mar
Prospective students and personal readiness assessment, 32–33
Print technology, 48, 66, 72, 127
Problem based learning (PBL), 132–133

R

Real Player, 40, 56
Reconceptualization, definition of, 59
  Clinical courses (see laboratory courses)
  Using a decision tree, 60–63
Required texts, 102
Responsibilities, students (see student learning
Rubric, definition, 147
Russell, Thomas, 3

S

Security, 51–52
Self assessment, 32–33, 42, 52, 83, 139–140
Self paced learning, 84
Simulation, 21
Storyboarding, 55
Student assessment, types of, 145

Initial assessment, 144
Continuous feedback, 145
End assessment, 146
Student learning
  Assessment (see student assessment), Characteristics of, 2, 16, 22–23, 113–114
  Expectations, 5, 115
  Responsibilities of, 22, 112–113
  Study strategies, 22–23
Student support, 31, 33
  Admissions and online assistance, 32
  Advising (see advising, students), 37–38, 42
  Career counseling, 37, 42
  Counseling services, 36–37
  Financial aid, 33–34
  Orientation, 23, 30, 42, 52
  Registration and online user friendliness, 34
  Technical assistance, 51–53, 56
  Technical requirements, 52
Student lounge, 131
Student tools, 104
Student tracking, 49, 51
Successful student characteristics, 22–23
Syllabus, course, 49, 101, 117–120
Synchronous communication (also see synchronous interaction, 129
Synchronous Interaction, 1, 4, 15–16, 21, 51, 92

T

Technical requirement, student (see student support)
Technological skill requirement, student (see student support)
Technology delivered instruction, 1
Technology needs assessment, 50
  Hardware, 50, 55–56
  Software, 49, 55–56
Technology in education, 20–22
Technology enhanced instruction, 1

Theories in education
  Behaviorism, 17
  Cognitive, 18
  Constructivism, constructivists view, 19, 80–82, 131, 139
  Social Cognitive theory, 18
Three click rule and navigation, 90

U

University of Phoenix Online, 106, 127

V

Video technology, 49, 66, 72, 127, 129
Voice technology, 48, 66, 72

W

Web based instruction, 1
  Best practice, 3–5
  Characteristics of, 1, 4–5, 15–16, 49
  Definition of, 1
  Vs. traditional face to face, 13–15
  Development (see reconceptualization)
  Evaluation of (see evaluation of course
  What's the difference study findings, 3
Web based learning, definition of, 1
WebCT® courseware, 40, 49, 52, 55–56, 94
Web Quest, 20, 89, 131–132
Web Initiative in Teaching (WIT), 93, 148, 152–163
Western Interstate Commission and Higher Education (WICHE), 31, 39
Where to start, 102

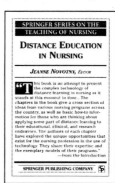

Springer Publishing Company

Internet Resources for Nurses, *Second Edition*

Joyce J. Fitzpatrick, PhD, RN, FAAN, and
Kristen S. Montgomery, PhD, RNC, IBCLC, Editors

Praise for the First Edition:

"The text transforms the morass of the Internet into a manageable, useful, and valuable tool for clinical practice."

—**Patricia F. Brennan,** RN, PhD, FAAN
School of Nursing, University of Wisconsin

New

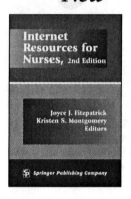

This new edition of the award-winning guide to the web for nurses is nearly double in size and twice as useful! Expert nurses in over 50 content areas have carefully selected and reviewed nearly 400 websites available in their specialty areas—resulting in an authoritative guide to the best the web has to offer for the professional nurse. Each web description includes a summary of the site, intended audience, sponsor, level of information, and relevance to nurses. Sites that also can be referred to patients are marked with an asterisk.

Partial Contents:

Part I: Professional Topics

- Professional Nursing Organizations, *B. K. Idemoto*
- Managed Care and Case Management, *E. V. Messett*
- Culturally Competent Care, *A. M. Villarruel*
- Returning to School: Graduate School Resources, *M. D. Fitzpatrick and J. J.Fitzpatrick*

Part II: Clinical Topics

- Consumer Health Resources, *C. A. Romano, et al.*
- Mental Health, *P. A. Wilke*
- Palliative Care, *J. T. Panke*
- Complementary and Alternative Therapies, *K. A. Guadalupe*

Part III: Evaluation Information

- Web Sites with Evaluation Guidelines, *G. L. Ingersoll*

2003   448pp   0-8261-1785-6   softcover

536 Broadway, New York, NY 10012 • Fax (212) 941-7842
Order Toll-Free: 877-687-7476 • Order on-line: www.springerpub.com